A SHOT OF

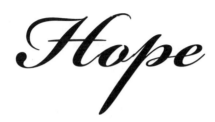
Hope

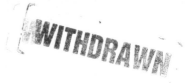

A SHOT OF

Hope

REAL WISDOM FROM A REAL SIBLING WARRIOR
PROVIDING REAL HOPE FOR AUTISM

ZACK PETER

Carrel Books

Carrel Books® is a registered trademark of Skyhorse Publishing, Inc.®, a Delaware corporation.

Visit our website at www.carrelbooks.com.

10 9 8 7 6 5 4 3 2 1

Library of Congress Cataloging-in-Publication Data is available on file.

Print ISBN: 978-1-63144-004-5
Ebook ISBN: 978-1-63144-020-5

Printed in the United States of America

CONTENTS

INTRODUCTION

"The siblings are our future," the lovely and inspiring Miss Jenny McCarthy spoke to a crowd one day. This woman has made such a social impact that she inspired me to become an advocate myself. "They are such amazing sources of love," she continued. "And one day, one of those siblings is going to write a book, and that book is going to change the world."

Well, my dear readers, that day has come. And *this* is that book (at least, I hope so).

Autism shakes up your world. It has changed my life and I wasn't even the one diagnosed with it, athough I did have an asinine science teacher in high school who asked me if I had been. Little did he know my actual story.

I do not have autism, but I am the big brother to, among five others, an incredible (and often mischievous) little boy who was diagnosed in 2005. His full name is Ethan Wolfgang, but we call him "Deets" (I'll explain why a bit later). He is one of the greatest gifts my family has ever received. And at times, one of the most challenging.

Because of Deets, I live a life that I never could have imagined. Starting at the age of sixteen, I've written a book, created the Play Now for Autism fund-raising brand, and hosted my own awareness-based talk radio show. It was all because my brother inspired me to make an impact on society. Now, as a young adult in my twenties, my life is nothing short of a blessing. But it wasn't always so easy. There were many early mornings, long days, and late nights. Some were frustrating, some lonely, some filled with triumph, and some filled with tears. This may sound shocking coming from me, a "self-loathing leech" (as I've been labeled online) who wrote a book titled *When Life Hands You Lemons . . . Throw Them at People.* But if there's anything this journey has taught me, it's that I do have a heart.

Autism truly has taught me a lot. It's taught me compassion; it's taught me the meaning of hard work; it's taught me the value of a sibling bond; it's taught me patience (which I have learned is very difficult). It's taught me how to make a really strong drink. It's also taught me how to hold on to hope, even when everything seems to be going wrong, when life has decided you could use a nice rainstorm right after making it out from under the tidal wave by the skin of your teeth. Don't act like you haven't been there, because you know you have. Everyone has. No matter how far you've come or what your life tolerance level may be, we've all been pushed past the point we thought had no return—the point we never imagined we could survive.

It has definitely been a journey. A long one that is far from over, that's for sure. When it comes to Ethan, he is not yet fully recovered. I'll be honest about that. He has his good moments and his bad ones. He never fails to amaze me, though. I am proud of him and so excited to see what the future holds for him, for myself, and for the rest of my family.

It's been a rough road with my family. Some of them support the treatment my mother has chosen for Ethan and others have been very against it, which has definitely caused some friction. But out of it all, life has gone on. *We* have gone on. I think that's one thing people forget: Autism doesn't stop your regular life from happening. It just adds to it.

I still grew up in a dysfunctional household, and had my own issues as a teenager, in addition to all of the advocacy-based projects I began to take on. When you take a very political world that feeds off controversy, and mix in a very politically *incorrect* kid named Zack, you have the perfect recipe for one emotionally unstable and slightly neurotic adult with a list of insecurities a mile long. But I chose to not let my brother's autism (or any other life challenges) break me. Instead, I allowed it to empower me. Now this is my journey of coming out of pity and using what I've learned to build a better life that includes a demanding career and a bright autism-free future for my brother.

I owe a lot to Deets. Every day I get to see my brother grow and improve; it brings joy to my life and makes all the struggles worth it. It's given me that spark of hope that miracles are real and they can happen to anyone, as long as you're willing to accept them.

The road is never easy and always brings strife. Sometimes you have to fight really hard to get to the middle, then try ten times harder than you thought you could to get where you want to be. Or at least somewhere near it. Sometimes, you really do need that drink at the end of a really long day, because Lord knows we deserve it (but less often than we think, I've learned).

So get ready, because this journey is a wild one. At times it will probably make you cry, but I'll do my best to keep you laughing. At times you'll smile, and at others I'm sure you'll probably gasp at some of the things I've had the gall to write. I'm nearly fearless because of autism. I'm not afraid to shake the ground. I'm not afraid to stand up for what I believe or against what I do not support. My hope is that by the end of this book, you too will walk away with an ounce more courage to keep going.

A SHOT OF
Hope

Author's note:

I have changed the names of certain persons in this account in order to preserve their anonymity.

CHAPTER ONE

The Game Changer

I was born with a mouth and an ounce of courage, and ever since I can remember, I've never been shy to use either. At the moment of my birth, my mother was ready to shoot me out, but I was just too comfortable in the water bed of her uterus and refused to be born. Which is why I put up a good fight as they vacuum-sucked me out of her. Basically, I've always put up a good fight when it came to a worthy cause.

I didn't have your typical "normal" childhood. Well, with the way things seem to be going nowadays, I guess it wasn't too out of the ordinary. The split household, the alcoholic stepfather, the busy mom, the love/hate relationship with food and dieting, the lack of direction or discipline, the nearly failing out of school—you know, the normal first ten years of a child's life.

Without getting into too much boring detail, my parents had me while they were still in high school, split at an early age, and after a couple years, they both got married again and started having more kids. So, most of my time was spent bouncing around from Mom's to Dad's, to Mom's mom's and Dad's dad's, but I was never really anywhere full-time. I assume this is part of the reason I can be so neurotic. There was a real lack of stability and guidance, so I kind of had to find direction on my own. And after a while I became very good at using my mouth and my ounce of courage to provide that direction for others. My mom refers to it as being "bossy." I just call it *making shit happen.*

Eight years after I was born, along came Ethan. It was March 2002. We had just arrived at the Huntington Memorial Hospital in Pasadena. For the weirdest reason, I loved it there. It was so big and empty and smelled a bit old, but still oddly felt full of life (or at least old people). I was so excited as my grandma and I walked out of the gift shop with yet another baby blue "I'm a Big Brother" T-shirt. Apparently three weren't enough. I jumped into the elevator as she flipped through the latest issue of *In Touch Weekly* featuring Anna Nicole Smith's latest diet trend. (This was before the Kardashians were on her radar.) I was just a few floors away from seeing Mom and my new baby brother, Ethan.

He was the cutest little baby. He was so chubby. My mom joked that he had eaten up all of her fat, since she had barely gained any weight during her pregnancy. I instantly felt a bond with Ethan. My other little brother, Elijah Joeb ("EJ"), who was just a year older than Ethan, was nothing but skin and bones. And very tan. You would've thought Mom had been sleeping with the gardener. Ethan and I were both lighter and much chunkier. Mom said he looked like me. Despite our having different fathers, he really did resemble me.

Ethan was my fourth brother. I thought that I knew what I was in for. And to be completely honest, I was right at first. Ethan was just like the last three little bundles the stork had dropped off. He giggled just as much, he mumbled just as much, and his dumps surely smelled just as bad. He laughed when I tickled him, he cried when he was fussy, he turned when Mom called his name. Everything seemed fine.

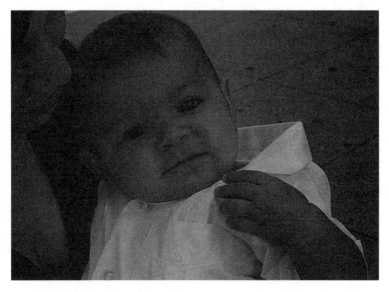

Introducing little Ethan Wolfgang!

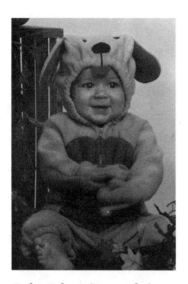

Baby Ethan (6 months).

Flash forward eight months.

"Deetens," EJ called out, trying his best to pronounce Ethan. Soon after, "Deets" became Ethan's new family nickname. "Deetens!" he continued to yell as Ethan looked out the window of our hotel room. It was bright and snowing outside. We were in Oregon on our way to visit family in Washington, which was a big culture shock from our home base in Los Angeles. Ethan just stared out the window, paying no attention to EJ.

Whatever, I thought as I ate my Cheetos and continued watching *Pokémon* on-demand. I didn't think much of it at the time, but something surely was a little different with Ethan.

My mom noticed it more than I did, as naturally a mother should. As I've gotten older I've heard her talk openly about having the initial feeling that Ethan may have been deaf, but almost certain that he wasn't, she searched for another possible answer. She says that something in her gut just knew it was autism.

It was shortly after noticing Ethan's withdrawn behavior that she called our family pediatrician demanding that Ethan be examined immediately. She knew that if she explained her "instinct" that it was autism, the doctor would likely put her off, especially since Ethan was still so young. So, naturally, my mother lied and said she believed Ethan *was deaf* and insisted that he be seen right away. The doctor dragged herself away from tending to her dying mother to take a look at Ethan. My mother felt bad for lying, but her baby's future was on the line. There's no stopping a mommy fighting for her child.

The doctor agreed that Ethan did indeed appear to have autism. The thing was, he was still very young. They couldn't really diagnose him until he was at least three.

I do not remember much about the day Ethan was diagnosed in 2005. I also do not remember anybody explaining to me why my brother had all of a sudden turned into a zombie. But I do remember Ethan before the diagnosis and his silly noises, how he would respond when I called him, and how he would laugh when I tickled him. It's funny how no matter how much time passes or other noises fill up our memory, there are always those special sounds that you never forget. That laugh was one of them.

There was a particular game I liked to play with him to get him to laugh. From one end of the kitchen, I'd say, "Deets! Ready? One . . . two . . . THREE!" as I ran toward him in his high chair. This would make him burst into peals of laughter. I was a natural-born entertainer and making my brothers laugh was one of the best feelings in the world. When I had annoyed all of the adults, the kids were the only ones who still paid attention to me.

Then, one day Ethan stopped.

It was like a light switch had gone off. That is the best way I know how to describe it. All of a sudden he stopped laughing at my kitchen games and my goofy faces. I'd tickle his stomach and he'd just sit there. No response. It was as if I didn't even exist. He was in his own world, and apparently, I wasn't getting the friend request. Or maybe I had just been blocked?

"Weirdo," I'd mutter as I waddled my chubby self over to play with EJ instead. It made me feel like I had failed, like I was no longer a good big brother. I didn't understand it. When I used the same bag of tricks with EJ or my other two brothers, they responded fine. But not Ethan. Sure I may have thought, *Weirdo,* but the real question in my head was, *Why is Ethan uninterested in me? I mean, I'm pretty hilarious.*

Autism was the last thing my family needed. My mother was busy with her job and raising her two newest little boys. She was also newly married to a man who she didn't realize had a strong dependency to alcohol that was only about to get worse. My father lived with *his* new little ones about thirty minutes away with *his* wife, managing a household of his own. Both parents were a little preoccupied and I hated to bother them. So having one more person who didn't pay much attention to me wasn't exactly helping my self-esteem. It just gave me another reason to eat that second gallon of ice cream.

I was a fat kid, and that's an understatement. A psychiatrist might say it was due to this household neglect, but it's also true that I loved food. And I had some nice, big love handles to prove it and a perky set of man breasts the kids at school wouldn't let me forget (as if I could really miss a pair that big).

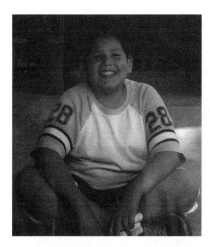

This was me, before I gave birth.

With everything else going on, receiving an autism diagnosis was not something my family was expecting. But hey, that's life throwing you a nice, big curveball.

By the time Ethan turned one, it was clear that something was different about him. He went from being a happy, typical-functioning, good little boy to a baby who basically just sat there. Something just wasn't right. I think we all kind of felt it, but nobody said anything.

Over the next few weeks, I remember overhearing mention of the word "autism." I was about ten years old and had no idea what the hell it meant. I thought it was spelled with an "O." As I regularly did, I continued to eavesdrop on my family's conversations to get the latest dish to later spill to my grandma, who paid me in Hot Pockets. Nobody sat me down to explain why Ethan was behaving differently. They were very matter-of-fact. I didn't like it when people kept me out of the loop. Still don't.

So, I took the one key word I had, sat my butt down at our computer, took a bite out of my Hot Pocket, and Googled it.

An abundance of complicated, confusing vocabulary popped up. *Great,* I thought. *More big words.* So I took it one click at a time. After about two clicks, I was so overwhelmed that I gave up. All I knew was that this "autism" thing had kidnapped my brother. And it sucked. More than the Nicole Kidman remake of *Bewitched*.

I saw autism as a bad thing. I didn't understand it. I didn't know what the hell it was. Nobody was talking to me about it, and the Google search was making pre-algebra look like a walk in the park. For weeks, I felt sorry for myself. I couldn't grasp the meaning of autism, but I knew it was one more thing that took my mom's attention away from me.

Growing up, she was my whole world. I was her first baby and she spoiled me rotten. I loved spending time with her. But after she reentered the dating pool, everything became about her new boyfriend, Jeff. Then they got married, had two boys, and were now juggling this asshole called *life*. It didn't seem fair. Then again, when is *life* ever fair? And then Ethan developed autism.

Our days soon became all about taking Ethan to therapy, making sure somebody always kept an eye on him, meeting with therapists and teachers, going on awareness walks, and watching Mom head off to support group meetings. They were support groups, not Alcoholics Anonymous. Though I would totally understand if she did go to AA. Just as long as she wasn't looking for her husband. Because he was hanging with his buddies down the street.

Autism can be a bitch. To a sibling, it really takes a toll. A lot of the extra responsibility gets heaped on us. But honestly, I would be lying if I said I wasn't happy to do anything that would make things easier for my mom and anything that would give me a little more time with her even though she was taking a lot of her frustrations out on me.

"I'm sorry, Zack," she'd tell me. "It's just that things with the boys and with Jeff . . . It's not fair to you, I know. And I don't mean to take it out on you. Don't worry, I'll make it up to you."

I don't know what it was that I wanted her to do. I just knew that there was an ugly wound inside me that I was hoping she could heal. I was consumed with a strong sense of sadness. I now recognize it as pity. I needed to snap out of it. And the only way to do that was to slap myself in the face and look at Ethan, a little boy who really needed a big brother. I didn't want him to have to struggle with learning how to figure things out on his own. I also didn't want EJ to grow up feeling neglected the way I had.

After a few weeks of feeling sorry for myself at the ripe old age of ten, I decided it was time to stop all the "woe is me" crap. If autism had kidnapped my Deets, I was going to go down to autism's house, knock open that door, and get my brother back. I was going to make sure I learned everything I could to find a way to save him. Nothing was going to stop me.

I sat myself down at that computer again and Googled like crazy until my head hurt. If there was any time in my life I wondered if I had dyslexia, this was it. I had no sense of how to organize the long words that floated past my eyes. I mean, did "autoimmune disorder" go before "deficiency" or after "candida"? What about "gastrointestinal tract" or "leaky gut syndrome"?

I remember looking up at my mom as she tore through book after book about autism. Sure she was busy, but her dedication empowered and inspired me. She was trying to learn as much about autism as she possibly could, and I was ready to be her wingman and do the same.

It wasn't easy and it took a lot out of me, but it was time for me to accept the cards life had dealt us and work with them. It honestly broke my heart to lose my brother, but I was determined to get him back. I had accepted my brother and accepted that this was the journey we were given, but there was no way in hell that I was going to *settle* for autism.

When a family member is diagnosed with autism, it's definitely a game changer. Autism hits you hard, like a train.

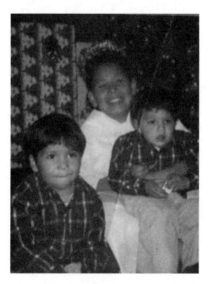

Look at my halo. I've always been such an angel.

And it can crush everything you have inside. I remember watching my mom sit on her bed at night and cry. I knew then in my heart that I was placed on this earth to fulfill a mission. Autism would become my key to unlocking that mission. It was time to pull out my sibling warrior cape and crush this train. And you can be damn certain that's exactly what I was about to do.

A Shot of Hope

The game is always guaranteed to change and likely at the most unexpected times. Just roll with it, and one day, you'll be so strong, not even a Trojan condom can stop you.

CHAPTER TWO

"Diet"

I t didn't take long before my mom jumped full force into mommy warrior mode, buying just about every book on autism she could find, researching every term, and attending as many local conferences as possible. She was determined (if only she was as equally determined to be on time . . . Sorry, Mom).

Her tenacity started to rub off on the rest of the family. My aunt got involved, my stepfather stepped up, and suddenly everyone seemed to be on board. Before I knew it, we were shopping at Whole Foods and Trader Joe's, buying nothing but gluten-free, casein-free foods, which are basically dairy-free foods, just a little more complex. Keep in mind, this was back when all gluten-free food still tasted like cardboard. Multiple sources my mom consulted indicated that putting Ethan on a GF/CF diet would help him—the theory being, many children on the autism spectrum have impaired digestive systems or allergies that make them highly sensitive to foods containing gluten and casein. I just heard the word "diet" and was hooked. My Slim-Fast shakes and nutritional classes weren't cutting it, and I didn't want to be the fattest kid in seventh grade. It might have helped if I didn't think a whole bag of chips was a single serving size.

My aunt thought my willingness to try the diet was stupid. She understood it more than I did. I just focused on the word "diet." Which the rest of my family seemed to focus on too. To me, diet meant weight loss. It's just how I associated the word. I often walked around saying I could eat only salads because I was on a diet. It seems crazy to look back at that now, being that at the time I was barely even a preteen. I shouldn't have been drinking Slim-Fast or even have understood what it means to "diet." That just gives you an idea of what kind of pressure I was under and the emotional turmoil I was trying to cope with at the time.

Having struggled with my weight for years, I had developed an ugly relationship with food and dieting. I was practically obsessed. To this day, I still struggle with it. But I've learned that people who tend to have these issues are usually feeling a lack of control in their lives. I was so used to being independent and on my own that I became a control freak (still am). When there was something in my life that I couldn't control, it affected my eating habits.

I often convinced myself that the less attention I demanded from my parents, the more attention they could give to my siblings. As long as they were taken care of and never had to experience what I did on a daily basis, all would be fine. I would take that bullet. This explained my obsession with being on a "diet." It gave me something to control in my life.

Other members of my family, however, interpreted the word differently. My grandparents were dead set against putting Ethan on a gluten-free, dairy-free diet. They pretended it was because they didn't understand the point or that it was too confusing to figure out what he could and could not eat. Since my brothers and I were often at my grandparents' house, my aunt printed out information for them and even put easy-to-read guides on their refrigerator. A gluten- and dairy-free diet really isn't complicated. Ethan couldn't eat wheat, cheese, butter, or milk, but he could eat meat, vegetables, potatoes, rice, eggs, and fruit. There were also gluten-free breads and other treats that could be substituted for the traditional options.

My grandparents fought constantly with my mother about this diet. Even my uncle chimed in, claiming to have done research that proved the diet was a hoax. I guess at some point he had gone off to study the human body and suddenly become a certified nutritionist. At least this was the way he acted.

"What you eat has no effect on the brain, Nancy," my uncle would tell my mother.

"Really?" she'd respond. "Take that logic to a bar right now and watch how alcohol affects how people behave. It's absorbed in the gut, goes into the bloodstream, and shoots up to the brain. It's the same with Ethan and gluten."

Go, Momma, I rooted quietly from the sidelines before coming to my mother's defense. "The diet works! Haven't you guys noticed how much better Deets has been doing?"

"Yes, Zack, but that's only natural. He's getting older. As he gets older, he develops. That's what happens. It has nothing to do with a *diet*," my uncle would respond. Sometimes he really pissed me off.

"I just don't get the point of putting him on a diet," Grandpa would add.

"Why can't he at least have a slice of cake at birthday parties? That's not right, Nancy," Grandma would add.

The house was like a war zone. Sometimes my grandparents would give Ethan food with gluten just to prove that it had no effect. I did not understand why everyone was so against it. If it would help Ethan, why not try it? Sure, the food tasted like dirt, but Ethan was young enough to get used to this new way of eating.

I didn't see it at the time, but their objection wasn't so much about the lifestyle change as it was about the word "diet." My grandmother even admitted to me that she didn't think kids should be on diets. To her it meant restricting someone from enjoying his or her life, the same way I associated it with weight loss and control. As for my uncle, I think he just didn't take my mother seriously. I just couldn't understand why anyone would try to discourage a mother from doing whatever she could to help her son.

It even became difficult with my stepfather at times. As much as he tried to be supportive of my mother, he still wanted to be the "fun dad." Just because cola didn't have gluten or dairy in it, he thought it was okay to give it to Ethan.

"That's a lot of sugar. He shouldn't have that," I would tell him.

"Well, it's not on the list of stuff he can't have. So according to your mother, it should be fine."

My stepfather and I didn't get along very well at this time, so I'm sure he thought I was just being a brat. That wasn't the case, though. I knew that a four-year-old shouldn't be drinking Coke, especially not Ethan, who would scream loudly and flap his arms like a flying monkey from Oz when he had too much sugar. I think it's insane that soda is an acceptable beverage at the family dinner table. Why not just feed your kids sugar straight from the bag?

Unfortunately, this struggle with how Ethan eats still goes on in my family to this day. In fact, I recently had a conversation with my grandfather about it, which began when he said to me, "So you get to travel the country and help kids with autism?"

"Yeah, it's pretty cool. I've seen kids who suffered from severe symptoms no longer having the diagnosis."

"That's good. So, what can we do for your brother? How can we help him? We should get him on this program."

"Well, the first step is the diet."

As soon as I said this, my grandfather retorted, "Well, I get it that it's a chemical imbalance, but I think there's something more we can do to help him."

I never said anything about *chemical imbalance*. The change in diet is about cleaning up Ethan's gut and healing his immune system. It feels like I'm talking to a brick wall sometimes. I wish my grandparents could understand the benefits of the diet for people with autism.

When Ethan was on a gluten-free diet, he became much calmer. Before that, someone always had to keep an eye on him, which was often my aunt or me. (My aunt was one of our greatest supporters at the time and I commend her for her dedication. She and my mother were true pioneers.) Ethan's entire mood was different when he ate better. Not only was he calmer, but he was more focused. He began using his words a lot more too. He also started to pay more attention to me. I never got his full attention, but I was no longer just a piece of furniture to him. Ethan was clearly improving. I don't care if my uncle believed it was simply because he was getting older. Bullshit. It was the "diet." He still clearly displayed symptoms in his development and behavior, but he was no longer such a zombie. It was as if the cloud around him was starting to clear. I was just waiting for angels to come out of that cloud playing beautiful music.

I remember the day Mom announced that Ethan's behavioral therapist noted he was a lot calmer. She said that he seemed more focused and was easier to work with. For some reason, this shit was working. People were beginning to notice it. For once, everything felt like it was coming together just as it should have been. Ethan was finally breaking free.

Honestly, at the time, I didn't fully understand what gluten or casein was. And I sure as hell know those GF/CF cupcakes tasted like they were made of grass and dirt. But hey, if grass-and-dirt cupcakes were helping Ethan, then I was all for them. It wasn't until after years of reading and interviewing doctors that I started to understand how the diet works. Now, I'm proud to say that I have chosen to live gluten- and dairy-free. Hell, I drink my coffee black and my vodka neat, so eating a diet free of gluten is no biggie.

A Shot of Hope

Don't knock something until you try it. Unless it's week-old sushi. In that case, please just walk away.

CHAPTER THREE

The Moment

There were times when Ethan would scream in a range about forty decibels too high. This was a common recurrence when he was upset or excited about something.

"What did he eat?" I'd mutter to myself, waiting for my eardrums to start bleeding. *What kind of "Coke" has his father been giving him?* Something was just off.

Normally, I'd just have to give him some attention and distract him with something else.

"He just needs to be spanked!" my grandfather would suggest.

"And what good is that going to do him? He's not going to understand why."

My grandfather's old-school mindset was that a simple pat on the butt would do the trick, but he didn't understand Ethan the way I did. I knew a spanking would probably just send Ethan giggling off into the other room, or worse: encourage him to injure himself because he thought he was bad. My uncle's solution was to give him more attention. "That's all he's looking for."

Ethan was seeking attention, but it wasn't just for attention's sake. There was clearly something wrong, something internally that wasn't adjusting well.

Sometimes I'd grab one of his essential oils and dab a little on the back of his neck to calm him down a bit. This was Mom's latest fad treatment. She had come across a woman who specialized in aromatherapy and decided to give it a try. It was helpful, I'm not going to lie. Ethan certainly did enjoy his oils. But by this point, I was ready to suggest that Mom look into medical marijuana as an alternative. I mean, look at the hipsters. They seem to be so chill.

Something had been more off than usual with Ethan, but I was having trouble putting my finger on it. And it's not like I had much help from anyone else in the family. Whatever my mother had tried to implement was taken as another silly attempt at pseudo-medicine by my uncle and grandparents, but none of them were offering any solutions. This is probably why I still get upset with people who are against biomedical treatments, like simple diet intervention and supplementation. Prescription meds do not always have to be the first choice. I don't understand why some people just don't get that.

Many of whom have the audacity to speak out without having tried any of the alternative treatments.

More and more, I noticed things were off whenever I babysat for Ethan. What everyone else had labeled as "typical Ethan behavior," I knew was not. Ethan didn't just throw tantrums for fun. He didn't scream because he enjoyed it. Clearly something wasn't right.

One night, Ethan, who was now about five years old, had been throwing a tantrum and was refusing to eat. I was angry and frustrated. It had been a long week. My stepfather was working late, Mom was off at one of her "meetings," and I had been suckered into babysitting. Again. Ethan wasn't happy because he had taken his *Thomas & Friends* trains outside to play in the mud and gotten them "all dirty!" So before I could get him to eat dinner, I had to make sure we washed them. Then, after washing them, he was upset because they were "all wet!" My patience was running thin.

I was desperately trying to get him to sit down and eat his dinner, but he kept crying and yelling. My head was pounding, my eyes were watering, and I grabbed the food off the stove and threw it on the kitchen floor, yelling, "God, Ethan! I just don't get you sometimes. Why does everything have to be so fucking complicated!" Then I broke down into tears, feeling guilty for snapping. I moped over to the couch, crawled into a fetal position, and began bawling my eyes out, hoping to wake up in the land of Oz. Or at least find some of Mom's Vicodin. (Kidding!)

At times like these, I felt like Ethan and I were on different planets. If you're a big brother like me, all you want to do is take care of your siblings. Sure they may piss you off more than any other human being, but you still always want better for them. That's the way I felt with Ethan. But with autism, this was beyond challenging.

I felt horrible, not only like I was a failure, but also like I was going crazy. I kept blaming myself for not having Ethan all figured out. I often put a lot of pressure on myself for that, which is the main reason nights like these were especially tough. Sometimes I just wanted to scream like Ethan. It seemed like a way to release everything building up inside of me.

Then, while I contemplated screaming my head off, I noticed it was quiet. Almost too quiet.

Oh no, he's on the roof, I thought as I began pulling my hair even tighter, making my face look more like Bruce Jenner's. Ready to drag myself out onto the roof, I finally noticed him standing in the doorway of his bedroom, looking right at me, and the guilt flooded every inch of me. Words can't even describe how horrible I felt.

"I'm so sorry, Deeties," I apologized for my outburst. "I'm really sorry. I didn't mean to . . ." I began explaining, realizing that my words weren't going to register with him anyway. My shoulders dropped as I stared at him. I didn't think I had any ounce left of emotion in me. Then something happened, something I never expected. I just looked at him and he looked at me, and there was a sense of understanding on both ends. We just connected on some deeper level.

People can have unique bonds with their friends and parents, but I think there's something special about the sibling.

You secretly can't stand each other most of the time but somehow still want to protect each other no matter what. You're each other's best friend, protector, and antagonist. It was a bond I felt was never quite complete when it came to Ethan. Sure, I felt like it was my job to protect him, and he surely knew how to antagonize me, but there was never really that sense of understanding between us. He was just in a different world. But for the first time as we both stood there looking at each other, I felt like we understood where the other was coming from.

"Hug?" I asked him, reaching out my arms. Then he walked right over to me and I started crying with him in my arms. Something clicked. We shared a tender moment of atonement. Ethan had never really hugged me before. I was so blindsided by what had just happened.

I felt like he understood that I was trying to help him and be there for him and that he was sorry for being a little pain-in-the-ass. To be honest, I really don't feel like this moment would have happened if it weren't for our attempt at putting him on the diet, this time adding in some essential vitamins and supplements.

This moment clarified for me that my brother was in there and he understood me. It let me know that we had opened up a little window inside of him and he was waiting to come jumping out. But there was still a lot more work we needed to do. It was this moment that empowered me to stay strong. Yes, I lost it and broke down, but hey, I was doing something right. Right? I mean, if I wasn't, we never would have shared this moment. And as tired and burned out as I was, I was ready to keep going.

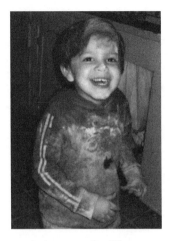

Let's just say he likes to keep us busy...

My mother said something once that made complete sense: "The more I learn about Ethan and autism, the more I learn about life." I love that quote of hers. It's so true. Ethan truly is a gift. I know sometimes I can speak about autism in such a negative light, but there is true beauty in darkness at times. Sure, I'm going to be the first to say autism is no walk in the park. It's not some beautifully wrapped package with a nice, big red ribbon on it that you open delicately. It comes in like Miley Cyrus on a wrecking ball, and you know what? Sometimes it just sucks. It's hard. It's really challenging. But I try to always at least focus on the good it's brought to my life.

I've heard some parents bitch, "What good?" What good? How about the strength and understanding it can teach? This moment taught me how to stay strong, how to fight, and how to hold on to whatever little bit is left in me.

Ethan never fails to bring challenges to my life. *That* I'm certain of. But now I've learned to love a challenge. Mainly because I know that after each obstacle, there comes a silver lining.

A Shot of Hope

Sometimes we're pushed so far past our limits that we snap. It's natural. I guess the best thing to do is accept and grow from it (with lots of really strong coffee along the way).

CHAPTER FOUR

Time for Action

There was one chilly day in Pasadena when Mom woke us all up early to make sure we were ready for our first autism awareness walkathon. I had never participated in a walkathon and thought it sounded exhausting. As excited as I was to be a part of it, I was equally dreading being physically active for an entire day. Mom loved being active. When I was in middle school, she used to try to make me go running around the neighborhood park before school. I don't think that lasted an entire week. Now her whole life had become dedicated to healing Ethan's autism, and this walk was an opportunity to get us all involved.

I wanted to help Ethan, so I agreed to participate even if it meant having to walk around the Rose Bowl all day.

We arrived clearly unprepared for the increasingly cold weather. It even started drizzling at one point. We walked down a long path from the parking lot to the actual event.

"Man, what a walk. Is that it?" I asked.

"No, Zack. We just got here."

"Oh," I replied as we walked onto the field and into the resource fair filled with aisles of booths. I, of course, hit up all the booths that were passing out free snacks. I even convinced a few vendors that I had a twin named Jack so that I could collect his seconds. "He can be really rude," I apologized. "I'll make sure it doesn't happen again. But I must tell you, we are triplets."

As we continued walking, I gathered information and learned about sensory issues and new therapies. I tried asking questions, but nobody seemed to take me seriously. They just smiled and continued on to something else.

"Geez, and I thought Jack was the rude one," I muttered.

After making our rounds through the resource fair, Mom dragged us out to start the actual walk, but not before she had hustled us a few more T-shirts. Can you believe they wanted us to raise a hundred dollars just to receive *one* T-shirt? It's a good thing my mother was swift with words. She can be a pretty good con-artist. Not to say I completely take after her, but I certainly have my way with words. If only my way with athletics was up to par.

"Oh my god, this is taking forever," I complained as we walked around the Rose Bowl loop.

"Oh, relax. We've been walking for only ten minutes," Aunt Abby snapped back.

Ten minutes felt like forever. Despite my mother's forcing me to play just about every sport as a child, I didn't enjoy anything athletic. If it involved walking or running—any type of moving, really—I just decided it wasn't for me.

We ended up completing the walk (with some sweat and a few tears) and left to go home for dinner. I collected just about every autism awareness pin I could find and proudly wore them to school the following Monday. My sweater was so filled with colorful pins, ribbons, and buttons that you would've thought I had mugged an old lady on the way to school. I was proud to be an advocate for my brother.

The walk became an annual family event for us. We tried to make it every year. It became so important to us that eventually Mom joined the planning committee. She had been working almost her entire life, but in the years following Ethan's diagnosis, she eventually decided that she needed to stay home and care for him, which paid off because he was really beginning to show improvements. With his therapies, his change in diet, and now Mom's constant attention, he was on the road to a promising future.

Meanwhile, I, now fourteen, was off trying to pursue a career in acting. It was something I had wanted ever since I was a toddler. I was such a natural entertainer that I knew I could build a career out of it. I would call up agencies and search for jobs on the Internet. I didn't think my mother took me seriously when it came to acting, but I knew no matter what that

I was going to make something of myself. And at the age of thirteen I landed myself an agent. A shitty agent, but an agent nonetheless. I've always been something of a hustla'.

So as I was off pursuing my acting career, Mom was back home taking care of the boys. I had just moved out of her house and in with my grandparents, which unfortunately meant that my life wasn't involving my brothers as much as it used to. Things with my stepfather's addiction weren't getting any better, and I needed to get away from it all. If my mother wasn't going to leave him, fine. I wasn't happy there, so I decided to leave on my own. And sadly, I didn't get much of a fight from her.

When I was fifteen, I left on a trip to New Mexico with my grandma one winter and ended up catching a bacterial infection on the way back (no, it was *not* an STD). I ended up having to see a doctor because it was getting really out of hand. I was breaking out in a rash all over my body. It was pretty disgusting. While sitting in the waiting room, Mom and I were flipping through magazines when the TV caught my attention. Usually TV always caught my attention, except when the news was on. But there was one story that really piqued my interest. It was about the Special Olympics.

"Kids with autism can play baseball?" I asked my mom.

"Well, those kids don't just have autism. Some have Down syndrome and other disabilities, but yeah, pretty much. There just aren't a lot of resources for them."

"Well, why not?"

"Most coaches don't care to take on the responsibility of having to manage a team that also includes members with special needs."

"Deets loves to play baseball, though. He always wants to run on the field when EJ plays."

"I know," she replied.

"Well, why don't we do something about it?"

"Well, what do you want to do?"

"We should host a baseball game just for kids with autism. We can call up all of your autism moms and get a game started at the park," I said, referring to the support group she had started calling Momma's Hope.

"Okay, let's do it," she said nonchalantly.

Mom was forever putting my brothers and me in sports. EJ loved playing sports, Ethan loved playing sports, and I loved eating Spaghetti-O's while watching *Jerry Springer*. So my idea of organizing a baseball game may have taken her by surprise, but hey, it was for Ethan. There weren't many resources at the time that allowed for children with autism to play on an organized team. Luckily for us, Mom always coached EJ's teams when he played sports. She sure knew how to trade in one hat for the other and kicked ass with every new project she took on. As long as she finished it.

Since Mom was the coach, she made up the rules and allowed Ethan to join EJ and participate during practices and in some of the games. Though he mostly just liked to run around the field and play in the dirt, he enjoyed being a part of the action. And he always loved to follow in EJ's footsteps.

Over the next couple of weeks, I continued to gather ideas for our baseball game. It was ironic that I was not a sports guy, yet I was passionately organizing this baseball game in honor of my brother. But that's the kicker: it was *in honor of my brother*. It wasn't about me. It was about being the sibling warrior I promised him to be. He needed me, and this was a chance not only to do something for him, but something for other kids too. For the first time, I was learning not just how to just care for someone other than myself, but also how to be truly selfless. There's no more rewarding feeling than being able to help someone else. After all, it wasn't Ethan's choice to have autism. It's not something he had any control over. It's just the card life dealt him. And though life had made things a little more challenging for him, I was going to make sure he still got to enjoy his childhood. But sometimes I got a little too ambitious and I thought I could outsmart life. That always ends well, right?

This baseball game became my main focus. My mental energy was buzzing. Then one morning, as Mom picked me up and drove me to school, it hit me: "We should call it Play Now!"

"Play Now?" She turned to me. "I like that. Play Now for Autism."

"Yeah! Play Now for Autism!"

And that was when Play Now was born. Mom then invited me to join one of her committee meetings, where I was introduced to everyone and shared my idea. Everyone loved it and told me how inspiring it was to have a fifteen-year-old taking such an active stance.

From then on, I was calling up parks, negotiating with directors, meeting with city council members for donations, and emailing potential vendors. In just two months I had pulled together what started as a small local baseball game and ended up becoming a full-on event. We were featured in the local newspaper, and I was even interviewed on the radio.

We raised a total of two thousand dollars at the event, which was all donated to autism research. It was crazy. My whole family came out to support us, even my father's side of the family. For once, everything felt like I was in the right place at the right time. And for teenagers, that feeling is rare. As a teen, you often feel like everything's a mess and everything hurts, and you have no idea how to control anything in your life. Your hormones are up and down and nothing feels right, but you constantly try to convince yourself that you have it all figured out. But for once, I felt like I had something figured out.

"You know, Zack, you should write a book. It would surely be nice to hear what a sibling has to say," one of the vendors suggested.

"Me? Write a book? Please. I can barely even write an essay and get a passing grade, let alone write an entire book."

"I think you should do it," my mom said. "Why not?" That's one thing I admire (and also find annoying) when it comes to my mother.

"I guess I can give it a shot," I said. Later that night, I went home and began writing. Within a couple of months I had what I thought was a pretty damn good book about autism. It shared different perspectives on autism and had lots of science, but not much of a real sibling perspective. I ended up finding a self-publisher, had my family pitch in a pretty penny, and got the book out there. I was young, had no idea how to publish a book, and had no guidance. *No guidance* was a recurring theme in my life. I always called the shots, and my family was always there to support me.

Later that year, the book was released, and I started hosting my own online talk radio show. I interviewed professionals in the autism and medical communities and covered provoking news stories. My life was taking off. Again, everything felt as if it was starting to fall into place. Everything was going so fast (and so well) that I just kept going. It was just so innate that I didn't really think about slowing down.

Eventually my high school got word of what I was doing and decided to make it a highlight on their website. Before I knew it, I was *that kid* who had written a book and done charity work for autism. Some kids were impressed, others were total dicks, and some continued to pretend like they didn't know me. Going in to high school, my goal was not to make friends or have an active social life. I was attending an all-boys private school, which I really didn't want to go to in the first place, so becoming popular wasn't on my list of priorities. I was just focused on getting my studies done and getting out of there. But as I got caught up in the activism, I realized that my impact was pretty powerful. Young people really can be amazing forces of change, and with a little direction, they can do really well. We just need to give them a little more credit. And a lot more slaps across the head when their arrogance takes over.

"I feel like I'm on a path," I told my great-grandma. "I feel like I started on this very wide path and I had no idea where I was going, but as I keep walking, the path seems to be getting more and more narrow, and it feels like it's heading in the direction it's supposed to be. The right direction for me."

"And you know what, baby?" she responded. "That's how God works. He has a plan for you. A big one. Trust Him. And keep going, my darling. And one day, your little brother is going to thank you. And I promise you, baby, he won't be the only one." It may just have been her cure-all of gin and raisins that had her in a good mood, but her positive vibes really rubbed off on me. And I was really looking forward to what was to come.

A Shot of Hope

When something feels right in your gut, go for it. You never know how high you can reach when you put your mind to something. And if all else fails, go talk to your grandma. If she's anything like mine, then she'll probably have a snack waiting in her purse. Just make sure it hasn't expired—#LessonLearned.

CHAPTER FIVE

Trolls

D espite my reluctance, as I mentioned earlier, I attended an all-boys private high school. My grandfather, my uncle, and my cousins had all graduated from this school, and I was next in line. I fought it for as long as I could until I just threw in the towel and went with it. It was either that or I would end up at the local public school down the street. I knew I'd probably be a lot better off at Cathedral High School than Gangbangers United. I'd also probably have less of a chance of getting shot.

Part of Cathedral's mission was to build strong leadership skills and instill a strong sense of brotherhood. We often had assemblies to help us learn how to better love one another the way Jesus loves us. It was Catholic, so the curriculum involved the teachings of Jesus. I personally have never underestimated the power of Jesus. In fact, he helped one of our instructors go from gay porn star to religion teacher, at least until the school found out and parted ways with him. But I'm sure he's off sharing his testimony somewhere more valuable now. Though, I don't know how much more valuable you can get other than at a school teaching young men how to become responsible adults. (#LessonLearned: Don't do porn.)

One day, we had a workshop conducted by a man who had brought himself out of poverty and gang life and into the world of motivational speaking, although I wondered if he was still on cocaine by his level of enthusiasm. I've done several motivational talks and stand-up performances myself, and I've never had that level of excitement. He was helping us build our brotherhood. I know Jesus teaches us to love one another how we love ourselves, but I'm sorry, it's hard to love a whole bunch of horny teenagers.

He made us all stand up together to make amends with one another. "Hug your friends!" he shouted. "Hug the men that you've had disagreements with! Go to them right now and make amends. Now is the time! Forgive!"

I looked around and thought, *There's gonna be a line around the gym of guys I have to make amends with.* Let's just say I wasn't the friendliest person in high school. It was also around the time my name started to surface in the autism community and when I got a clear idea of how cruel people could be on the Internet. I was experiencing a little dose of what is known as *trolls*: Internet bullies with nothing better to do with their lives than bash people for not agreeing with their (most of the time) biased points of view. They're kind of like crabs, just way more annoying and harder to get rid of. Hey, maybe we can create a vaccine for that? Pharma, get on it! I see a big moneymaker here.

The trolls gave me the bullying experience I had never experienced in my actual high school. Since I never shared any of this with my family, I didn't have anyone to comfort me through it. And since I already had an abrasive mouth, I didn't let anyone mess with me. So let's just say I didn't have many friends. Or really any at all.

I decided not to participate in our "making amends"/forgiveness fest. I just sat there and watched all of the other students hug each other and work through their issues. I didn't care to make any friends, and I was not in the mood to begin working through my issues with my classmates. As it was, during our breaks and lunchtime I often spent my time taking calls regarding my first book, or podcast, or the events I was planning. Or I was finishing up homework I hadn't done the night before because I was working. I used work, and a number of other things, as a distraction to keep me busy and not thinking about what I was going through emotionally.

I had young siblings I needed to protect. I had a mom I needed to help. I even stood up for my dad when my mom wanted me to ask him for more child support by telling her that he had other kids and a wife to provide for. I took on a lot without finding a place to release everything I had snowballing inside me. This was one of the reasons I didn't want friends. I didn't have an ounce of emotion left to invest in friends.

So I sat there all by myself as I watched everyone around me participate in this love fest. A part of me wanted to barf, while another part of me wanted to crawl into a ball and hide. I acted like I was too good to be there, but inside I was ready to break down. So I just sat and waited for the whole thing to be over, praying that if Jesus really did love me, he would expedite this process.

In the middle of my boredom, one large, bear-sized student walked over to me. I had never had much contact with him but often saw him around campus. He was a defensive lineman on the football team, and if I'm being honest, they weren't the sharpest tools in the shed. They were still tools, just more like hammers: dull and hardheaded.

He walked over and looked down at me. I pretended to not see him standing over me. That wasn't very believable since he blocked any light that came from that direction. I would also be lying if I said a part of me wasn't desperate to fight my pride and turn to see what he wanted. It could've been one of two things: he either wanted to atone for making some stupid joke about me behind my back, or he wanted to borrow a buck for lunch.

"Oh, come here, bud," he said to me with his arms wide open.

Oh brother, I thought. I would rather give him *two* dollars than dare to participate. But something urged me to stand up and embrace his act of kindness. It was very thoughtful of him to walk over and acknowledge me. Especially since I don't think we ever spoke more than five words to each other.

If I wasn't an emotional wreck before the hug, I was one after. It wasn't bad enough that only *one* person decided to acknowledge me, it was the one person whom I didn't even know. I was just about ready to bawl my eyes out, but instead managed to thank him and wait for the whole shindig to be over.

Following the assembly, we went back to class. I tried not to give it another thought.

There was a group of seniors who enjoyed heckling me as they walked around campus, calling me names like "Peter Penis." I had caught them bullying one of my classmates one time and didn't really appreciate that. Sure, I wasn't very active in social activities with my peers and only talked to them if I needed to copy their homework, but one thing I never allowed was for bullying to take place in front me. This had put me on the seniors' shit list.

Anytime they saw me, they'd whisper to each other while staring at me and laugh. I'd ignore it because the whole thing was rather pathetic. They were older yet acted like mean girls in a movie. They weren't anything special, and I made sure to remind them of that as often as I could. It was really only two members of the clique who really didn't like me, but I added them all to my own shit list anyway.

One of them walked up to me after school on the day of the assembly. I was not in the mood to put up with his little pussy-posse and immediately put my guard up, assuming he had something stupid to say to me. We had just received our year-books but I doubted that he was coming over to ask me to sign his.

"Hi, you're Zack, right?" he asked.

"Yeah."

"The one who does the work for autism?"

"Yeah, and . . . ?"

"I just wanted to know if you'd sign my yearbook?"

"Why would you want *me* to sign your yearbook?"

"I think the work you do is very courageous, and I'd like you to sign my yearbook."

I looked right at him and said, "And why do you care?" I thought it was a joke. I thought at any minute his little gang was going to come out of hiding and laugh at the prank they were trying to pull on me.

"I knew someone who had autism," he told me.

"Oh," I replied. "Did they die?" I bluntly asked him. He used the words "knew" and "had," so I just assumed that this person had passed away.

"No, actually . . . they recovered." And that was the moment my foot shot straight into my mouth, my heart dropped to my stomach, and I felt like such a complete and utter jerk. I was the biggest jerk to this guy. The word "recover" instantly told me this guy knew what he was talking about. Most people use the word "cure" and somehow discredit it while bashing Jenny McCarthy, who's been so public about autism and the available treatments she used for her son.

"Oh . . . Wow. I'm really glad to hear that," I said as I signed his yearbook.

"Yeah, thanks," he said with his head down before taking his yearbook and walking away.

I was speechless. A part of me wanted to run after him and apologize profusely, but I was frozen. I felt awful for being rude to this kid who actually looked up to me.

Later that night I sent him a message on Facebook apologizing for my behavior. I explained how I assumed that it was all a prank and that I was sorry for my attitude. Then I asked him who he knew had autism. This is where I officially won the title "Douche Lord of the Year." He told me it was him, but thanks to treatment, his autism had improved.

Slap me in the face and screw me with a cactus. Here I was, trying to be a voice for families and people with autism, and I had just been the worst possible person to a young man who had received a diagnosis himself. This was when I vowed that no matter how difficult the road ahead of me had become, I would never again allow myself to become heartless to the people around me. It was one of the most humiliating and humbling experiences I have ever had. To this day I cringe at the thought of it.

I've surely made a lot of mistakes, but one thing I learned was that I needed to defrost my heart a little bit. I know I can come off as very snarky and maybe even a little mean. I'm honest to a fault, but one thing I never like to do is hurt anyone's feelings.

This happened in my junior year of high school, the same year I decided to leave Cathedral and complete my senior year through an online homeschooling program. I needed a little break from people and wanted to focus on myself and on my work in the autism community. The environment I was in wasn't very healthy for me and I needed to get away, so I moved from the center of Los Angeles to a slightly more suburban outskirt, hoping to really be able to refocus my attention in the right direction.

A Shot of Hope

There's really no cure for trolls. Just throw some bread crumbs while keeping it moving over the bridge they live under.

CHAPTER SIX

Charity Bites

I was only sixteen when I got my first real dose of the cut-throat world of charity. Following the success of the first Play Now event, I decided that I wanted to keep organizing fund-raisers for autism. I enjoyed doing this, and it kept me busy.

I joined my mom in supporting one of the most widely recognized national autism organizations around. We served together on the planning committee of the organization's local annual walkathon. It had become a family event for us, so volunteering felt natural. I was still only a teenager at the time, so everyone seemed so impressed that I wasn't as much concerned with taking selfies as I was with actually trying to have some sort of positive social impact. As much as I love attention, I knew that there was more to this world than myself. I loved donating my time to the cause, and my craving for knowledge grew. I wanted to learn everything I possibly could about autism and share the knowledge with as many people as I could. To me, everyone in the autism community was on the same team fighting for the same cause. Little did I know that politics were apparently a lot more important than the cause itself, at least to some people.

When I decided to continue organizing fund-raisers, I began exploring other services being offered by other organizations. I didn't want to stay glued to just one. I wanted to branch out and use my voice in as many places as I possibly could. My thinking was this: my brother can't speak, and neither can many others like him, so I'll be their voice. My intentions always were and always will be entirely pure. I enjoyed providing a place where kids with special needs could come together to participate in sporting activities and feel free to be themselves without any judgment. And a place for their parents to allow them to play freely without getting the "evil eye" from other parents who don't have children with special needs. You know, that look that just pierces through your soul and makes you feel like the worst person in the world? I used to be intimidated by it when I was with Ethan. I remember when Ethan would throw a tantrum smack in the middle of the supermarket. Next thing I knew, we'd be surrounded by people giving us the evil eye. I've now learned to wave and pose for pictures while they stare. Or, when I'm really not in the mood, I'll just flip them off. Not that flipping off a group of people in public is courteous, but come on now, is it really necessary or helpful to stare someone down when he's clearly embarrassed enough as it is? I wanted to create an environment for parents of special-needs children in which they could feel understood rather than judged.

The money raised from my first fund-raiser had gone to an organization that seemed to be doing a great job at generating awareness and donating money to research. But this time around, I wanted to work with an organization that offered services and support to the families directly. I sent in an email inquiry explaining my idea and detailing the success of the event I had previously hosted. After a couple of calls and emails, I officially had a new beneficiary for the event.

In the weeks leading up to the event, I thought a good way to promote the event would be at a mixer that was being hosted by the group for which I was a committee member. I thought they would be excited to see me branching out and getting the word out there about autism and generating support in the community. There would be a lot of families in attendance, some that had come out to last year's Play Now event, so this would be a great opportunity to get the word out about this year's fund-raiser. I thought it would be a nice win-win situation.

Well, the man in charge of putting together the mixer didn't like that idea. He ended up sitting me down and explaining that there was a "conflict of interest" in supporting another organization. To me, that made absolutely no sense. Who cares where the money was going? It was an event for families. *There were families here.* It was an event that benefited families. *These families would benefit from the support.* It was made very clear to me that if I chose to support another organization, I would no longer have the support of this one.

Initially, I was taken aback by it all. I didn't think I was doing anything wrong. I still clearly had plenty of support from both organizations (multiple ones, actually), it's just that I had chosen to donate the proceeds collected from a fund-raiser to an organization that had assured me the money would go directly to supporting a family in need. To me, when there's a family in need, there's never a conflict of interest. Besides, it's a *charity*, not a damn presidential election. Politics and picking sides should have nothing to do with it.

My mom agreed that it seemed odd and unfortunate but made sure I didn't get too discouraged by it. Yes, it was upsetting, but it wasn't worth getting worked up over it. And since I technically wasn't allowed to promote my fund-raiser *inside* the actual mixer, I decided to gather my flyers and place them on all the cars surrounding the venue. Don't allow me to give out my flyers during your event? Fine. Tell me that if I support others I am no longer welcome on your team? Not so fine.

I proudly walked away from this particular "conflict of interest" and never looked back. And I'm very proud to say that I have been supported by a long list of other autism organizations since then, and all have been completely fine with all of my "conflicts of interest."

I did also lose a lot of good "friends" in the process. Ironically, as time went on and my departure became known, I began losing a lot more "friends" and "supporters." The organization even went so far as to put my closest friend's job in jeopardy for this friend having supported me. (Yes, I do have at least *one* friend.) Who does that?

I've never been one to keep mum about what I believe or where I stand on things. I think social media is a great avenue for this. Even though a lot of people use social media irresponsibly (myself included), it's still a great place to network, share ideas, and create a platform for social engagement, as I began to do. Some people were very supportive of me. Others bashed me for it. Coincidentally, they happened to be strong supporters of the group I had left. I began receiving a lot of backlash for my beliefs, one of which is that environmental triggers may have been a contributing factor to my brother's autism, which I still firmly hold to be true.

I was instantly labeled as "anti-vaccine" even though I'm not. But I do believe they should be administered with a little more caution. Perhaps they should be spread out a little, instead of given all at once. Or there should be more research on whether mixing them creates any serious side effects. I wished that people would just relax with all of the online crucifixions. The hate tweets and brutal emails were stupid and served no purpose. These people weren't saving the world by attacking a kid on Facebook, let me tell you.

As a seventeen-year-old trying my best to do the right thing, I began spreading what I had learned about autism, information on potential links and triggers, and helpful treatments and therapies. A lot of this stuff had worked for my brother, so I put it out there. Well, the more I put out there, the more flack I got. It was another case of the trolls.

I've had some of the most horrific things said to me, like my brother was made for natural selection, or that I use him to make money. To this day, I donate portions of my earnings and continue to donate my time to this cause and to the recovery of my brother. People should be lifting each other up and sharing what we've learned, not bad-mouthing each other.

There were these two older men on Facebook who would constantly try to put me down. Both of them were fathers of children on the spectrum, and both of them were major jerks. I couldn't post a single thing about autism (or anything, really) without their trying to discredit me. It's as if they enjoyed trying to make a seventeen-year-old look stupid. When I posted the cover of my second book, which had a photo of my pulling my hair and yelling at the top of my lungs with my mouth wide open, one of them even had the nerve to comment, "I especially like your fangs. They give the cover a nice touch."

All of the negativity was really starting to make me not only question myself and my motives, but become more and more disconnected from people. I no longer trusted my friends and didn't even want to share things with my family. I felt very much on my own, like I was no longer fighting a battle for my brother, but now having to defend myself. I even began questioning whether or not I was worth defending, or if I really was a bad person for choosing to step up.

This entire journey as an advocate for my brother and for this cause has been tough. Criticism on any level is never easy to deal with. Let alone when it's extremely negative, condescending, and just plain cruel. But I've learned a lot from all of it. I've gone from fighting off the online trolls, to taking on too many projects at once, to running my own failing business. When I was seventeen I wanted to create a line of T-shirts that would raise awareness about autism. The proceeds were to be donated as well. At seventeen, you don't have the tools or knowledge to handle running a business on your own, especially while still trying to finish high school. Needless to say, it burned up in flames right in my face and left me in debt for quite a while. I've dealt with numerous "haters." I once got into a mini-Twitter feud with Penn Jillette of Penn & Teller fame over vaccines. And sometimes I've made really stupid decisions and put my foot in my mouth more times than I would like to share. But I didn't let that discourage me either.

I'm still very young, but I've been around the block quite a few times. I may not have *all* the answers (even though I often pretend I do), but let me tell you, I'm not going anywhere. This is my mission. This is my heart. This is my brother. Nothing will ever come between that. Nothing will ever knock me off my game, even when the players like to bite. Guess what? I can bite too. That's what these "fangs" of mine are for.

A Shot of Hope

"Haters" and critics are part of life. Whether they're high school students or forty-year-olds who should know better, they're not going away. The only thing that can go away is your negative outlook. And if all else fails, you can always just flip them the bird and keep walking.

CHAPTER SEVEN

Hope for Recovery?

Mom and I were in the car driving back to my grandmother's house. I had recently decided to officially move in with my grandparents after things at Mom's had gotten a little too crowded, and, to be honest, I wasn't very happy there anymore.

"*Mother Warriors*? What's this?" I asked my mother as I held up a white hardcover book in my hand. It had a photo of a woman with short blond hair and a child who appeared to be her son.

"That's Jenny McCarthy. She wrote that book," my mother replied.

I had heard the name before but never really knew who she was. I often confused her with Jennie Garth. In fact, when

I found out Garth was going to be on *Dancing with the Stars* I told my mom (thinking of McCarthy) because she was such a big fan.

"A nation of parents healing autism against all odds," I continued to read off the cover. "Wait, so she found, like, a cure for autism?" I asked, intrigued. "This is huge. You mean, we can cure Ethan?" I didn't factor that if there was a cure, it would likely be too expensive for us anyway.

"Not exactly. She doesn't refer to it as a cure. There is no cure for autism . . ."

"Yet," I interjected.

"Right. *Yet*. But Jenny's found that by making changes in diet and with detox she has healed her son's autism. And when you heal someone's autism, they'll never be fully cured, but they'll be *recovered*. Think of it like being in an accident. You can recover from that, but you aren't technically *cured*. You can get better and improve your condition, but you'll never fully be the same as you were prior to the accident."

"That makes sense," I agreed. "So can we *recover* Ethan?"

"Well, with the GF/CF diet and other applied biomedical treatments, I'm sure we can. But you know how tough that's been."

"Yeah, I know," I replied, reflecting on how reluctant everyone around us seemed to be to sticking to a simple diet.

"Why don't you take the book and read it. I think you'll really like it," my mother suggested, even though I wasn't really one for reading. I'd always had difficulties focusing on a book, at least until I found this one.

I took the book home and began reading a little bit every day when I got back from school. I was shocked to see profanities in a book and that it was not only inspiring, but actually pretty funny. I didn't know books could be so unorthodox. That's one thing I admire about Jenny—she is far from orthodox. I would normally procrastinate getting started on my homework by watching *Maury*, but reading this book seemed like a much more appropriate pursuit.

In reading *Mother Warriors*, I found hope. I learned that recovery is real; it just wasn't being shared enough. There was so much information out there that people needed to know about. There was a whole group of parents called warriors, and they were healing autism! The book mentioned Generation Rescue, a nonprofit organization providing resources and hope for autism. On their website it says, *Hope for Recovery!* It had stories of families that were successful in healing their children. They even had a grant program for low-income families that would help jump-start the treatment process. I couldn't believe that this was real, and sadly, not as commonly known as other autism resources.

I'm going to heal Ethan's autism, I promised myself. *I'll make sure he gets to do all the things other kids his age get to do.*

When it comes to healing autism, there are lots of mixed emotions. I've found that some people are very supportive of the idea and others are very against it. The way I see it, it's not necessarily about changing a kid. It's about giving him a better life. Sure, it's nice when your brother gets enrolled in a great school for children with disabilities and lands in a great class for kids with autism. But I didn't want Ethan to have to be in a *special class*. I wanted him to be in a *regular class* in a regular school. He has the potential. Why not try to help him excel? If a "typical" kid struggles in school, what do people do? They hire a tutor, get him extra study time, and maybe cut out some of the extracurricular activities. If a kid is diagnosed with ADHD, you might give him some medication or change his diet and basically do whatever you can to ensure that he does well in school, right? So, just because there is an "incurable" medical diagnosis for the child, why does that designate that child for a "special" class? How about getting that child help, addressing his medical issues, and working toward his overall educational well-being? That doesn't sound too out-of-the-box to me. You're not "changing" the child. You're aiding in the child's success.

Sure the argument can be made that children with autism are special children and should be treated as such. But guess what? Every child is special. Just because there is a medical diagnosis doesn't mean you should handicap the child. Allow him to live to his fullest possible potential.

I was curious as to what services Generation Rescue offered. If this resource was what had helped Jenny's son as well as other children, I certainly wanted to learn more about it.

After meeting the Generation Rescue staff as a volunteer, I began to ask more about the grant program they offered and what a family might need to do to qualify. At that time, candidates should not have received any biomedical treatment other than dietary changes. The family's household income had to be within Generation Rescue's qualifying range. Luckily for us, we were in that range and all we had tried with Ethan was changing his diet.

"Hey, Maddie," I asked the mother who ran the program one day. "What exactly does the grant program do for families?"

"Well, it's basically a jump start to treatment," she explained. "We give families a supply of supplements and vitamins, strategies for diet intervention, appointments with certified doctors who are trained in treating autism, lab testing, and other support to help guide them."

Wow, I thought. *This sounds awesome!* This was just what Ethan needed. "So how would someone apply for a grant?" I asked.

"Well, you have to take a placement test to determine where you're at, meet the qualifications, and you must fit within a certain income bracket based on where you live. If all of that checks out, you can apply."

"This is what I should get for Ethan! Do you know how much he can benefit from it? And you can apply for your niece, too," I told my friend Lina soon after. She had a younger niece with autism and would often join me when I volunteered at any of the benefits or fund-raisers for the cause.

"I don't think my sister would go for it," she responded. She seemed so disinterested, almost as if it wasn't that big of a deal. Hel-lo! Improving autism over here! How is that not a big deal? I don't understand people like that. If it's available to you, why not try it? At the very least, *try* it. And I'll tell you right now, try it we surely did! (Look at me, talking like Yoda now.)

I filled out our Autism Treatment Evaluation Checklist, got my mother's household tax papers, filled out the application, and turned it all in to Maddie. She reviewed it, went through the normal application process, and the following week we were approved for the next round of grants. It was so exciting.

We received digestive enzymes and probiotics, vitamins and supplements, a daily logger, lab tests, and a physician to help us get a customized protocol in place. Maddie even agreed to be a mentor to help guide us (I put her on speed dial). Ethan was taking a multivitamin, omega fatty acids, enzymes, therapeutic supplements, methyl-B12 lollipops, and remained on a strict GF/CF diet. It was crazy to see how much calmer and more verbal he was becoming.

We even set up an appointment to visit a trained physician who would help us figure out what approach to take with Ethan. And thankfully, Ethan was having one of his bad days when we arrived for our appointment. As I've previously described, Ethan would occasionally have these little bouts during which he would get giddy, laugh uncontrollably, scream, and just act out. His behavior was just out of control. I figured taking him in like this would give his doctor a clear picture of what was going on and help him lead us in the right direction.

When we arrived at the doctor's office, there were toys laid out in a section of the waiting room that was just for kids. I hoped that Ethan would settle down and play with the wooden abacus. But there was clearly something going on inside of his body that was not reacting well. We now needed Ethan not only to behave, but also to sit still so that he could be examined. I'll tell you right now, Ethan was not about to have *any* of that.

After seeing Ethan's hyperactive behavior and restlessness, his doctor concluded that he clearly had way too much yeast in his GI tract. Yeast overgrowth is usually caused by too much sugar, like, say, too much soda. Also, I learned that if Ethan consumed too many starchy foods and wasn't active enough to burn off all the carbs, his body would turn it into sugar, which then manifested itself as yeast in his gut. This discovery was huge! It explained so much. But I knew once the rest of my family found out that Ethan now had to reduce his sugar intake, it was not going to go over well. Remember "fun dad" and "restricting him" from enjoying his childhood? Yeah, now let's take away the sugar. I'm sure they'll understand, right?

I, personally, *love* sweets. And I know how much Ethan loved his sweets, especially candy and soda. This was something my immediate family would have to tackle head-on, but it was going to take some time to ease everyone else into it. I couldn't believe everyone else's acceptance was beginning to take priority over Ethan's health and overall well-being. But it's just how things had to be if we were really going to do this.

Ethan really did show amazing improvements after beginning the grant program. Again, he was calmer and so much more focused, especially after taking his vitamins and supplements. Ethan, who had been almost entirely nonverbal (with the exception of a few repeated words here and there), was now beginning to say full sentences. He went from having what seemed like a more moderate degree of autism to a more high-functioning autism. He still clearly displayed autistic-like symptoms, but they were subsiding.

I remember being over at Mom's house for dinner one night. My stepfather Jeff, who at the time was studying culinary

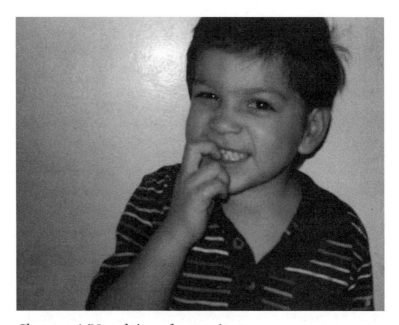

Cheeeeese! (Non-dairy, of course.)

arts at Le Cordon Bleu, was cooking dinner. We were his guinea pigs, and he loved to make us new dishes. He served Ethan his rice and fish with a side of some veggies (butter-free, of course).

"Is that good, Ethan?" he asked.

"Mmmm, yes! I want more, please!" Ethan said, as we all smiled, appreciating the milestone. I couldn't believe it. It seemed so surreal to be at a point I thought would take years to reach. It was nothing short of a little miracle that would hopefully mark the beginning of a new journey.

A Shot of Hope
All things come in their right time. Patience is the key. I just can't always find it when I need it.

CHAPTER EIGHT

Florida's a Beach

In 2011, I received an invitation to speak at an annual autism conference in Florida, partly thanks to the support of a woman named Kim Stagliano. As a mother to three daughters on the autism spectrum, she has put a tremendous amount of work into helping this cause. She has also helped me spread my message.

I often joked that Mrs. Stagliano and I were involved in a romantic relationship and that she was my cougar girlfriend. Real girlfriend or not, Kim has always supported me, and landing this speaking engagement was a huge deal. It was my first real presentation at a national conference. I had spoken to small support groups, at local events, and to students, but never at a conference. Never had my name been listed as a featured speaker on such quality-grade paper.

I was excited and immediately shared the information with my mom, who agreed to join me on the trip. It would be my first big work trip outside of California. Naturally, my mother wasn't going to skip having some steak and beer on the beach . . . or supporting her kids, of course. I asked her to book the flight and she said she'd take care of it.

When I looked at the departure/arrival times, I noticed that we were flying out on Thursday afternoon and weren't flying back until Monday evening. I needed to be there only Friday and Saturday and had planned to be home by Sunday evening.

"You booked us for two extra days," I texted her. She claimed it was an accident, and since they wanted to charge us two hundred dollars each to make any changes to our itinerary, I figured it was best to just keep it as is and try to enjoy the extra time together. After all, we were going to Florida. Who wouldn't enjoy a whole weekend on the beach?

When we arrived at the hotel, I decided to head down early to find the room where the conference would be held. I walked around for twenty minutes trying to find the damn room. All the arrows that pointed to where the room was supposed to be kept leading outside. Finally my mother joined me in this quest to find the hidden temple, and one of the hotel staff members pointed us to a hallway in the corner of the lobby. We walked over to the hallway only to find yet another exit.

"What, did they put us in the parking lot?" my mother asked.

"That's what it looks like," I responded.

We walked out the door to find another door outside that led to a conference room. It was a good-sized room, just extremely difficult to find. I scouted the room, trying to imagine it full of people in their underwear, but this wasn't helping me overcome any nerves. I decided to go for a walk to calm myself down.

When I headed back to the conference room, I assumed there would be about fifteen people tops. I was surprised to see it overflowing with people eager to hear my perspective as the sibling of an autistic child. As if I wasn't nervous enough.

When my session started, I introduced myself and then read an article I had written for *Age of Autism*. It was a collection of my thoughts on what it was like to be a sibling mixed with little bits of advice for parents, such as the following:

- Parents, acknowledge your kids! *All* of them. Even if there are twenty of them.

- Set a day out of the week, or month, that you can use as a day to spend with your neurotypical kids. Show them some TLC. Set the day and please keep it. My mom left a lot of false promises of Mom-and-Zack days that I didn't see much of growing up. It killed me. Don't do that. It's bad karma.

- Help them understand autism. Talk to them about it. Get them involved in the advocacy. It makes them feel "in the loop." Bring them to your meetings. And don't lie and say you don't go to meetings or conferences. You do. A lot. I know. This is bonding time you can use, so use it.

- "How do I get my kids to understand autism?" you ask. Don't buy them Holly Robinson Peete's book. Just kidding! But seriously, those books are a dime a dozen. And nothing beats one-on-one time with YOU. But if you're going to buy them a book, don't just hand it to them and say, "Here, honey, read it." You read it first so that both of you can discuss it. And if your kids come up with an idea for a family outing or something that involves participating in your family's advocacy, don't shoot them down. Embrace it.

- "How do I connect with my 'typical' kids?" Who do I look like? Oprah? You can connect with your kids by, again, spending time with them and *just them*. And be sure to tell them that you love them many times. Even if they beg you not to. Deep, deep down, they like it.

- "My kid wants no part in the advocacy. What do I do then?" you ask. Buy him a sports car. All right, that might not do much, but I sure wouldn't mind getting one for my birthday (wink, wink, Mom). Really, if they seem disinterested, don't force anything on them; it'll just push them away.

- Don't *always* make them babysit. They'll most likely agree to do it, but try not to put them in this position too much.

- Keep them involved, but don't overload them. Remember, they're just the siblings, not the parents, so having them change diapers, babysit, rub your feet, cook dinner (not necessarily in that order), make you a margarita, and then clean the walls after they've been written all over might be a little too much to ask.

Following that, I did a Q&A with the audience and gave away some free stuff, which is always a crowd pleaser. I was really shocked to find that most of the questions parents were asking they already had the answers to. They just weren't trusting that what they were already doing was enough. I provided my perspective and gave them some advice as to what they should be doing and how to involve their other children. They seemed pleased with my anecdotes and my insight, which helped me feel more confident. It also didn't hurt that they found me very funny. I like it when people find me funny.

After wrapping up with a few more questions, I thanked them all for coming and invited them to my book signing the following morning. I then went back up to my room to get some well-needed rest.

The next morning I headed off to my book signing. That also went better than I had expected. In fact, that morning I had brunch with the president of the organization.

"So how do you feel it went?" she asked me.

"I think it went really well. Better than I thought it would."

"Good. How would you like to return next year?"

"Really?" I asked. I expected this to be a one-time, wham-bam-thank-you-ma'am kind of thing. I didn't think they'd really invite me back. Apparently I had done something right. "Yeah, I would absolutely come back!"

"Perfect. So I'll mark you down as the first speaker to return next year," she said with a smile.

I was stoked. The rest of the day my mother and I spent exploring the hotel and enjoying our time on the beach. This trip would've been a perfect two-to-three-day thing. I wouldn't have even minded taking a red-eye out that night. I actually like red-eyes; they get me where I need to go and back in a timely manner, leaving extra daytime to do other stuff.

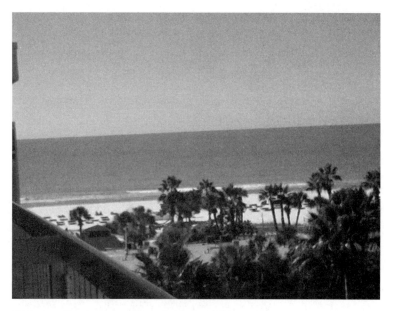

This is what we were saying good-bye to.

The day after I got back from Florida I had to attend an awards ceremony at the Beverly Hilton. I was nominated for the Outstanding Youth Volunteer award for my advocacy efforts.

I ended up taking the award home. Sure, I had worked really hard and endured ridiculous circumstances, but receiving recognition for doing charity work just felt unnecessary. I was extremely appreciative, but I didn't really *need* the acknowledgment is what I'm getting at. The Florida trip had really worn me down, but that was just how my life was as a result of becoming an activist. I didn't hate it, but I was quickly learning how demanding it could be. Not to mention that as

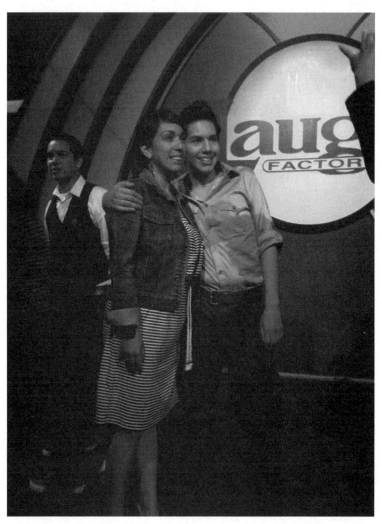

Nancy and me.

soon as the awards ceremony was over, I was called in to do a temp job with another charity for the weekend. I ended up spending the weekend at my grandmother's and continuing to live out of my suitcase from my Florida trip. What kept me going was that working for charity is one of the most gratifying experiences a person can have. It's one thing to write a check, but to actually get your hands dirty and put in the hard work and know that you're helping to better someone else's life— that's true philanthropy.

A Shot of Hope

Work hard. Unless you're a Kardashian. Then just sell a sex tape and you're set for life.

CHAPTER NINE

Catalina Island

I apparently hadn't had enough travel time with my mother because I agreed to go on another trip with her four months later. Her birthday is only a day before Ethan's, and with EJ's birthday only a week later, we usually celebrate all three birthdays at the same time.

"We're going to Catalina Island for our birthdays. Want to go?" my mother asked me.

"Sure," I agreed. How could I tell her no? I had never been to Catalina Island, and I thought this would be a good bonding experience for the four of us. Ethan was turning ten and EJ was turning eleven, so they were at a good age to be able to enjoy a trip like this.

The day we were set to embark on yet another adventure, however, I found out that it wouldn't just be the four of us. The trip would also include two of her friends, her friends' kids, and one of her friend's boyfriends, along with his young daughter. We would end up staying in two hotel rooms, one of which would harbor the children—the room I happened to be assigned to. Their ages ranged from four to eleven. So not quite the moody-teenage range, but still in the bouncy/hyper/answer-my-million-questions age range.

After checking in, we walked down to the local liquor store to buy snacks for later that night. The boyfriend bought a bottle of tequila, which I assumed was preparation for some sort of party he was planning to throw. Or maybe he was an alcoholic who couldn't go a single night without consuming an entire bottle of alcohol. Either way, unless a clown was on his way or the boyfriend was willing to dress up to entertain the children, I wanted no part in whatever was coming next.

"So are we still going out later?" Friend One asked.

"Yeah, we'll see," Friend Two replied.

Already I didn't like the way this was turning out. First, I was blindsided as to whom we would be traveling with. Second, I was catching on to the fact that I was not just a participant in this trip, but the elected babysitter for the evening and possibly the entire weekend.

"We might be going out tonight, so the kids will be staying with you," my mom told me.

"Well, thanks for the heads-up," I said monotonously.

Ethan wasn't feeling well, so Mom decided to give him some cough relief syrup and put him to bed. It was also around the same time the rest of the kids fell asleep. Despite the fact that I wasn't really tired, it was night-night time for me too. Meanwhile, all of the adults went out to some club named after a woman's breasts. Luckily, the first night turned out a lot smoother than I was anticipating.

The next day, the kids all woke up early and were eager to play. We started off at a park down the street. Following that, we decided to grab breakfast and set off on an adventure throughout the island, which is just what some of the adults needed to work off their hangovers.

We rented bikes. Everyone got his or her own beach cruiser, while I got a dual bicycle that I shared with Ethan. I didn't think much of it when I volunteered, as I assumed a dual bike worked the same as a single-person bike.

As soon as we took off, I found that riding this bike proved to be exponentially difficult. The second I kicked off, the bike began leaning to the left. I managed to get us down the road before I concluded that the bike was messed up.

Maybe I'll just shift my weight, I thought as I began leaning to the right, which sent us tumbling over to the opposite side.

"What the hell," I muttered.

"What's wrong?" my mom asked.

"This bike. Something's wrong with it."

"Here, let me try it." She experienced the same level of difficulty, if not more. My mother is much shorter than I am and she isn't very muscular (not that I am either).

"Here, don't ride it. I think I'm just going to take it back," I told her. That's when I noticed what appeared to be the culprit: Ethan. You see, a two-person bike needs *two* people pedaling.

When only one person pedals and the other one just shifts his weight around, the bike tends to lean and this makes for a very challenging ride.

"That's what it is," I announced.

"What?"

"It's Ethan. He's just kicking back, enjoying the ride."

"Oh Deets," my mom said, laughing it off.

"All right, Deets," I said. "You need to pedal. You need to help me push the bike. Okay?"

He looked up at me like I was speaking French, then turned and began enjoying the view of the beach. I hopped back onto the bike and was determined to catch up to everyone else. I kicked off and hoped for the best.

It took about three whole seconds of my hair breezing in the wind before Miss Daisy and I went tumbling into an innocent little girl, smashing her ice cream cone.

"Hey!" Ethan yelled at me.

"Hey? Hey buddy, I need you to help me or else we're going to be crashing into everything. Okay?"

He gave me a dirty look and got back on the bike. We then set off once again.

"Push, Ethan. Push! Pedal, pedal, pedal," I kept repeating.

Finally after I had learned how to balance left to right, alternating between my weight and Ethan's, we were able to set off to find the others. We decided to take a shortcut and went riding right through the caravan of tourists in front of us, dodging little girls with ice cream cones and not minding the sign that read, No Bikes beyond This Point.

Between avoiding people and cars and cheering Ethan on, we were able to make it safely to the rest of our clan, which had barely even noticed that we had been MIA for the past thirty minutes.

"Let's go up the hill!" one of the kids shouted.

"Yeah, let's go," they all began cheering.

"Ugh," I moaned before pushing off toward the big hill. Everyone else had sped off while Ethan and I huffed and puffed behind. "Come on, Ethan. Push! Pedal, pedal, pedal," I said, trying to keep my breath.

When he continued to disregard me, I stopped pedaling. As we began to lose our balance, he shouted, "Hey!"

"*Hey* back. Come on. We gotta move. This choo-choo train is running out of gas and I need my caboose to get going."

He finally really started to haul it up the hill. We pushed and pedaled as hard as we could. We were like the Little Engine That Could, but we really, really didn't want to. The others were in the distance, and we were desperate to catch up. We were just a little more than halfway there when we saw them one by one passing us back down the hill.

"Motherfucker," I muttered.

"Motherfucker," Ethan repeated and laughed.

"No, no, no! Don't say that."

"*Don't say that!*" he mocked.

"Ethan."

"*Ethan.*"

"Stop."

"Motherfucker!" he blurted out again, laughing.

"You know what, you're right. *Motherfucker*," I said, sharing his carefree attitude. "Let's go back down." What was the point of spending another thirty minutes going uphill when we could just glide back down and still be fully caught up? Not that anyone noticed how far behind we were.

I assumed riding back down would be easier, as we weren't going uphill. I was wrong. The increased speed made for a much more challenging ride. I thought having to carry Ethan's dead weight up the hill was a struggle, but having to break with Ethan's dead weight was even tougher and led to a few more tumbles. Not to mention that the whole way down, Ethan was singing, "Motherfucker, motherfucker, motherfucker," and laughing hysterically. I had no more energy at that point. If it was socially acceptable for me to join him and sing along, I would have done so.

Ethan and I decided to part ways with the rest of the group and head off in our own direction—a direction with a lot more flat land and still a few *more* tumbles.

During our nice joyride around the island, I noticed that we seemed to be going in circles. The same houses and the same school we had seen three times were becoming less and less amusing. That's when we learned that Catalina Island really isn't that big and there aren't very many things to see. Finding the beach was actually anticlimactic. Living in LA, I had seen lots of cool, hippie beaches. This was really nothing new.

"All right, Ethan, we need to find them. This trip is wearing me out."

I don't know how we lost our party on such a small piece of land, but of course, with our luck, they were nowhere to be found. I wouldn't have been surprised if they were off having dinner somewhere. It was starting to get dark and my legs were hurting. I knew if I was getting tired, Ethan must have been, too. Just when that thought crossed my head, Ethan threw in the towel and gave up pedaling, which sent us into a full cartwheel onto the pavement.

"Oh shit! Motherfucker," he muttered, which piqued the attention of passersby, who were shocked to hear a ten-year-old curse.

"Yeah, he said it," I yelled at the people watching. "What are you going to do about it?"

Even more mortified by my rudeness and lack of authority over Ethan's potty mouth, they gasped and walked away. I couldn't care less. Ethan was merely saying out loud what I was thinking in my head. Most people find it so offensive when kids with special needs curse. You know what? I'm just happy that my brother can say any words at all. I don't care what words he chooses, as long as they express how he's feeling. Is it a little embarrassing at times? Sure, but I'd rather him say the F-word than be completely nonverbal. One thing I admire about my brother is that he doesn't have a filter. He's just who he is completely. I respect that.

Just then I saw half of our group ride right by us. As Ethan picked pieces of gravel out of his knees, I picked him up along with our bike (and any bruised dignity we had left) and began dragging the whole lot. They kept riding. We could've been lost, or eaten by some sea monster, or possibly even kidnapped by pirates, yet nobody seemed at all alarmed. If I would've known that, I would've parked our bike an hour ago and taken

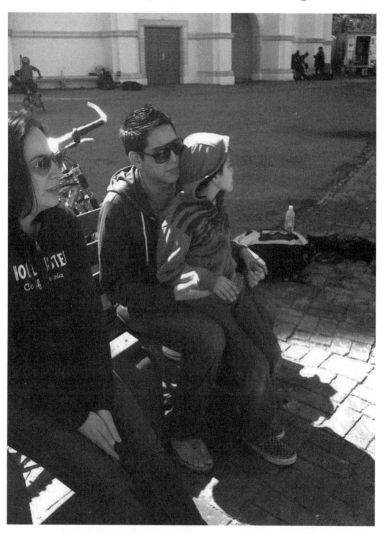

Ethan and me on Catalina Island, taking a break from doing cartwheels with our bike.

Ethan for some sorbet and souvenir shopping. Lord knows that would've left us less injured physically and emotionally.

It was on the boat ride back to normal civilization that I found out that my first two books had appeared in the top three spots of Amazon's bestseller list.

"Oh my God! My books are number one and number three on Amazon!" I exclaimed as I began showing everyone my phone displaying their ranking.

"Wow, that's awesome," my mother told me.

I sat back down, looked out the window into the pitch-black ocean, at Ethan, and then back out the window. I had a sense of peace. This meant one of two things: my life was going right according to plan . . . or I just passed some gas. Either way, it felt pretty damn great.

Ethan, like any little brother, can drive me crazy at times. But for some reason we were put together in this eccentric herd that we call our family. And though they drive me equally as crazy at times, I'm glad I have them. They help me stay grounded, they always support me (when they don't forget about me), and they keep my blood flowing. And, of course, it doesn't hurt when after the madness you can add bestselling author to your résumé.

A Shot of Hope

Laugh. Laugh at yourself. Laugh at the absurdity of your circumstances. Just laugh. A lot. And appreciate that you can have a sense of humor about things. Not many people can do that. And if you can, you're already #Winning. Oh, and never go on a trip with my mother.

CHAPTER TEN

Falling Off the Wagon

It was a warm summer day, and I was in the car with Mom. Not even fifteen minutes previously, we had been at her house with my stepfather, all sitting on the couch watching a Whitney Cummings comedy special on Netflix, laughing like one big happy family. *Things seem to be falling right into place*, I thought. *Man, who would've ever thought that things would finally start to look up.* Then she said it. "That's my new apartment. We actually just drove right past it."

"Your new apartment?" I responded, a little thrown off. Why would they move from a cozy house to an apartment? And why would she call it *her* apartment?

"Yeah. I'm moving out. I already have my own apartment. I'm moving in next weekend. You should come over and help me move all my stuff over. It'll be fun."

"What?" I responded, so confused. "What does that mean?"

"Well, Jeff and I talked, and we've decided that we want to be happy and maybe this is the best way to do that. We're still going to be friends. And we've already talked to the boys about it."

I sat silently. I didn't know what to say. I didn't know if I should be mad, or upset, or happy for her, or . . . *What about Jeff?* I thought. *Am I ever going to see him again?* Growing up, I nearly hated Jeff. But by this point, I'd started to really look up to him, like a real father figure.

What about the boys? What about Ethan? How is he going to react to this? Change does not go over well for kids with autism. They don't like it. Shit, I hate it. And I'm considered "typical."

It wasn't fair to the boys. It wasn't fair to Jeff. He clearly still loved my mother very much. It seemed like this life she had fought so hard for was now slipping away like a balloon in the wind, and she was letting it fly away. I didn't know how to respond. The remainder of the car ride was pretty quiet. I just didn't know what to say.

But she seemed so calm about it. Almost . . . *happy*? I hated for her to be unhappy. But, Jeff used to make her happy. How could things have changed? I just didn't understand it.

Part of me was really upset, because no matter how ugly things got between them, she always fought to make it work. Many times I felt like she had chosen him over me, that making her marriage work was more important than whether or not I was happy living with them.

I had been gone for only a year, yet so much had changed. I imagined how Ethan and EJ must have been feeling. Here I was mourning the separation of my mom and my stepdad, but for my brothers, this was the end of their mom and dad, pretty much.

I began to reflect on everything up until that point. When I had decided to move to a more suburban outskirt of LA, Ethan was well into the grant program, leaping full throttle into recovery. He was speaking a lot more, and he was a lot calmer. He was doing well. Things really looked up. Now, everything was starting to slowly fall apart. How can things be fine one minute and changed the next?

A few months went by and things seemed to go along steadily, at least for Mom. Her new apartment had come together pretty well. Things with her and Jeff seemed fine. The boys didn't seem to be affected too much by having to split their time between Mom's apartment and Dad's house. But I could tell Ethan's recovery was falling on the list of priorities. Within the first year, he had really regressed. He wouldn't really say words as much as he would mutter and grunt them. He seemed a little angrier and distant. And how could I ignore his drawings when I babysat him? They were of two houses with four people, one that read Mom, one that read Dad, one that read EJ, all under a sun with a sad face. I remember bringing it up to my grandma, who also seemed concerned by it. It was clear that Ethan was having a tough time.

"I don't know what to do," I told my grandma over lunch. We had just left the Laugh Factory in Hollywood, where I had had a meeting for the first Laugh Now for Autism comedy benefit. We walked across the street and ate at this really nice, but really small, Italian restaurant. Things for me seemed to be coming together nicely. I was performing at the Laugh Factory with the comedians of Chelsea Handler's talk show, *Chelsea Lately*, and in two more months, I'd be hosting the third annual Play Now for Autism event. I had just recovered from my failed clothing line and everything for me, personally, was looking up again. Now how could I fix things for my mother and the boys?

"I don't know," my grandma replied.

"I mean, growing up, I felt like she wasn't really there for me. And I never demanded any more attention from her because I wanted it to go fully to the boys. But I mean, come on, what is she doing? Ethan doesn't seem to be doing any better. And those drawings? I just wish I knew what we could do," I contemplated with her.

My grandma seemed just as confused and defeated as I was. I could see the hurt in her eyes. She continued to tell me about how horribly Jeff had been doing since the split. How he had been drinking more and how he came over one night and poured his heart out to my grandfather and her. I could tell she was hurting for Jeff just as much as she was hurting for those boys. But I was no longer seeing them all on a regular basis. I felt like it was so out of my control. I was beginning to feel really guilty.

Before I knew it, my mother was moving out of her apartment and in with a good friend who also had kids. In addition to the boys dealing with two households, they now had to share one of those households with another family. All of Ethan's biomedical treatments went completely out the window. He began eating pizza and hamburgers and drinking soda. It was getting bad.

I had just started my second semester at college when I decided that things were just getting too out of hand. I knew it was time to put my mommy issues aside and start working on a better relationship with my mother. I began having dinner every Thursday night with Mom and the boys. It was nice, but Ethan would always act up. He would yell and would run around the restaurants. He would jump into other guests' booths and sometimes drink their sodas. I was very uncomfortable, to say the least. I wanted to speak up, but it just didn't feel like my place. I was his brother, not his parent. There was only so much I could say. And I didn't want to embarrass my mom in front of everyone. I would try my best to settle Ethan down but made sure to not step over any lines. That was one of my biggest challenges.

I love my mom and my brothers, but sometimes dinner was just so unsettling I got anxious and embarrassed by how badly Ethan was behaving. A couple of times I even broke down as soon as I got home. I knew internally that Ethan wasn't well, which was manifesting itself in these behaviors. To see my brother not doing well and feel paralyzed is one of the ugliest feelings I've had to encounter. I felt completely defenseless. And then to have to watch my mother, the one person who used to be the head force of everything, now just sitting back and allowing this was unbelievable to me. What was happening to her?

"Why don't you just move in with your mother?" my good friend Calvin told me one day.

"It's not that easy," I replied.

"Well, you said nobody's doing what they need to for Ethan, so why don't you?"

"Back it up for a minute, okay? It's not that easy. You're forgetting, I have a job, I go to school, and I have several other projects that I'm running here, not to mention a weekly show that I host, write for, produce, and help edit. I can't just give up my entire life for this. As much as I desperately want to, it's just not that easy. And I really don't need you to make me feel any more guilty than I already do. I cry at night over this. You know that. We've talked about this over and over. It's not easy for me, but I'm not Ethan's mother. I'm not Ethan's father. There's only so much say that I have in all of this. It kills me to feel like I haven't been there enough for them and that it's my fault that Ethan's regressed. I blame myself for not being there enough as it is. But I have to accept the reality that it's his parents' responsibility. There's only so much I can do. I can give them everything they need, but it's up to them whether or not they want to enforce it."

"No cheeseburger! No *cheese*burger!" I remember Ethan demanding one night because his burger had arrived without cheese. So my mother then asked for another burger, but this time *with cheese*. "No *milk*shake!" he yelled, and my mother ordered him a milkshake. What about the gluten-free, dairy-free diet? It was completely out the window.

I was even more baffled when we went to a Dodgers game and he put some soda into his sugary, blue ICEE and finished it! This was followed by candy and a Dodger dog. I could not believe it. When he ate like this, he would not only yell out his demands, but he'd take his clothes off and run around. Then there was his laugh. It was loud and uncontrollable and haunting. It was like he was doped up while drunk at the same time. His eyes were dead like a drug addict's.

"Are you seriously going to let him eat that candy?" I asked my mom. "After everything he just ate?"

"Well, I wasn't the one who gave it to him," she replied, sounding defeated.

It was like she had lost the fight that once burned so strongly within her, the fight that inspired me to get so involved. When looking back at the past couple of years, I got it. It made sense. She now had to provide for these boys on her own. She no longer had the stability of having a husband or a full family household. My family was completely unsupportive of biomedical treatment for Ethan. I was now no longer there as much to help her stand strong against them. She had fallen off the wagon and there was nobody there to help her get back up.

"I don't get it. It's like she can be so fucking selfish sometimes," I told Calvin one evening at dinner. It was the day after my cousin's birthday party, where all day I was chasing Ethan around the park, making sure he wasn't sipping any stranger's soda, or taking his clothes off and laughing, or running too far away. I was so angry and frustrated and tired. I was busy, I had a pretty full plate with work, and I wasn't expecting to be the only one watching Ethan. At age eleven, Ethan shouldn't have needed anybody watching him.

"I just don't know what to do," I continued. "It hurts to see him clearly hurting. It just makes me so mad that nobody is doing anything for him."

"Look, Zack," Calvin began. "I know how much you care. I know how much you want to see Ethan get better. *I* want to see Ethan get better. But you know your mom is clearly not where she should be. Her mind isn't where it should be. Your family isn't on track. So if nobody's doing anything, somebody has to. That somebody has to be you."

Calvin was right. That somebody did have to be me. But the truth was, I didn't want it to be me. Don't get me wrong, despite the fact that some of my family members often expected my mother to fail, I was always cheering from the sidelines for her to prove everybody wrong. It's not that I couldn't fight the fight; it's not that I couldn't win the battle to help Ethan. It's that I didn't want it to have to be me. That may sound a little selfish, but I wasn't meaning for it to be. I wanted it to be my mom. I wanted, at the end of it all, when the boys were both old enough and well enough to look back at this time in our lives, to say, "Wow, Mom. *You* did it. *You* healed Ethan. Because of *you*, everything is all better."

Maybe I was manifesting something from my own childhood. I had really felt completely thrown out the window the second my

stepfather came into the picture. In the earlier years of their marriage, things weren't pretty between them. I kept waiting for my
mom to leave him and take us out of that environment, but she
never did. I just kept waiting for her to step up and fight for that
little boy named Zack who was really unhappy and needed his
mom. Maybe, in my attempt to make sure my siblings received
better treatment than I did, I was somehow using the pain from
my own childhood to put more pressure on my mother to do
better for my brothers. That seems logical, right?

In all honesty, with Ethan's recovery, I wanted her to be
the one to receive the acknowledgment. I believed in her. I was
still rooting for her. But Calvin was right. Somebody needed
to step up and do something. Somebody needed to be the
one to intervene. In my heart, without Calvin having to say it,
I just knew it had to be me. This was my mission. I don't know
why, but this was it. Ethan gave my life meaning. He gave me
purpose. I owed it to him to give every bit of my power and energy. He helped me find this courage and strength, and now it
was my time to use it. See, I was good at fighting in the autism
community, but now I needed to fight within my own family.

If Mom had fallen off the wagon, so be it. I was going to
help her get back on. If my family wasn't on track, so be it.
It was my time to step up to them. And I did.

"So what's going on with Ethan's recovery?" I asked my
mother at dinner one night.

"Well, we want to get him back on the GF/CF."

"So why haven't you?"

"It's just been tough. Nobody's willing to support it. Nobody believes in it."

"Well, you just have to convince them. Lie to them if you have to. Tell them you took Ethan to the doctor and he was tested for food allergies. Tell them Ethan's allergic to gluten and dairy. They should believe that. Dramatize it if you have to."

My uncle had had a bad allergic reaction to dairy and after going to the doctor, it was determined he had some severe food allergies. Suddenly everyone had become very cautious and aware of his dietary needs, which just seemed so contradictory to me, as they hadn't supported Ethan's. So I figured this was the best time to work off my uncle's situation by saying that Ethan also had food allergies. It was true, so it's not like we would be lying to them. It was just a matter of convincing them and getting Ethan's diet back on track.

"I know. I have to get back on it," my mother said.

"But you have to be strict. I can get you everything you need to help him, but I need to know it's not going to waste."

"Well, if you can get it, I'll make sure it gets some use."

As promised, I got her everything she needed. I got Ethan all his supplements: his omega-3s, his multivitamin, his digestive enzymes, his supplements for all the yeast that was clearly in his body. I made sure I read and reread *Healing and Preventing Autism*. It is by far the bible for healing autism. It has everything you need to know. If there is any book you should read on autism and treating it, this is the book. It's written by Dr. Jerry Kartzinel and Jenny McCarthy and is the best book

I've read on autism. I asked my friends at Generation Rescue about what we needed to start over. I was fully charged and ready to rumble. This was it. This was Ethan's time to finally get everything he needed. Now it was just time to get everyone on board. All aboard the Rescue Train!

A Shot of Hope

If at first you don't succeed, try and try again. Eventually you're bound to get somewhere, right?

CHAPTER ELEVEN

Holi-daze

Mom was now back on track and fully prepared to make sure Ethan received the proper treatment for his autism. It was tough, but she was making baby steps that were slowly becoming big-girl steps. All she needed was to recharge her battery and she would be back on fire.

Being around my extended family during the holidays proved to be a little challenging, however. Normally we would go to my great-grandmother's house, where most of my mother's side of the family would gather. The house wasn't very big and there were a lot of us. Personally, I didn't like going over. I didn't really have much in common with most of my cousins, and I got anxious trying to make sure Ethan didn't get yelled at. This was also the side of the family that believed "Ethan just needs a spanking." Ethan didn't have the ability to stand up for himself. *Yet.*

I told my mother I didn't want to go, but she convinced me to after we agreed to have dinner at her house first so that we didn't have to spend the entire night at my great-grandmother's.

"What time are we going over?" I asked my mother.

"Probably around eight," she replied. It was a little earlier than I was hoping, but it was Christmas, I wasn't in a bad mood, and I was actually looking forward to our annual game called "White Elephant," which is when everyone participating brings one wrapped gift (usually a gag gift), which we put altogether in a pile, and then in random order, we select one of the gifts to open and take home. It was always fun to see what people ended up with. However, it was finding something gluten-free, dairy-free, and sugar-free for myself and Ethan to eat that was sure to be the real challenge. I'm a huge sugar junkie so I always like to keep treats out of sight for fear of going overboard. My mentality is basically, *Well, I already ate two, so I might as well just finish the entire box.* But hey, it was Christmas. It was the time of year you're allowed to get fat and just hide your love handles under an oversized sweater.

Of course, at 7:45 P.M., my mom says, "Okay, we'll leave right now. I just have to wrap these gifts," as she begins putting gift after gift on the table. I exhaled through my nose loudly as I helped her do what she should have done two hours ago, when she spontaneously decided to bake cupcakes. But that's my mother. She's the type who'll wait until fifteen minutes before we're supposed to leave to get ready, and then all of a sudden decide to bake a cake. This drives me crazy.

We stopped by my stepfather's house to pick up EJ and Ethan. When I saw that the boys weren't ready, it suddenly made perfect sense to me why my mother had married Jeff. His time management skills were just like hers.

"Wow, dude, you really grew up!" he told me.

After he and my mother split up, I rarely got to see him. I noticed he had a couple of beers in him.

"I know, and you . . ." I started.

"I know. I'm fat now. But hey, would you ever trust a skinny chef?"

"Probably not," I said, as I laughed with him. He then went on to show us what he had made for dinner. He's a damn good chef and gets to travel the country working all the A-list celebrity events. The only thing was, his cooking didn't look very gluten- or dairy-free.

He read off the menu he had prepared for the boys. "They're all fed. Ethan's been in and out of the kitchen all night picking. And I know, the potatoes have cheese, but . . . oh well."

Oh well, I thought. *It's just your child's health.* I wanted to say something, but I just let it go. It was Christmas and not the time, nor the place, to go there.

It was clear to me that even though my mother was on board with Ethan's biomed treatment, I still had some work to do. This was also the moment I really empathized with her. Not only did she not have my family's support, but my stepfather wasn't exactly fully on board either. He was more like having one foot in, one foot out, but with autism treatment, you need to have both feet chained to the center of the boat.

I had given many kudos to Jeff in the past for the way he had really transformed his life. To be completely honest, I was even leaning more toward his side when I found out their marriage had ended. Initially I was upset with my mother, but as time went on, I really began to understand her side of it all. And in the past two years, she and I had gotten a lot closer. Making Ethan's recovery a mutual focus really brought us back together.

Mom had gotten the boys squared away, and we were ready to go. Now that we had Ethan in the car with us, I was starting to ache a little more in my gut. I knew there would be lots of foods and sweets Ethan couldn't have, not to mention all the soda and how congested the house was going to be. Ethan's sensory and dietary needs were surely beginning to worry me.

Upon arriving, I found myself a seat near my grandma and uncle by the beverage table. A few minutes later, Ethan walked into the room and immediately wanted soda. *Here we go*, I thought as that gut feeling began to worsen.

"Come on, Ethan," I said. "We don't need that. It'll hurt your tummy. Let's get you some juice." (Juice that I fully intended to water down.)

"Why aren't you going to let him have that? Just give it to him. He wants it," my uncle said in a slightly condescending tone. With my grandma watching right beside him, I knew the second I even dared to respond I would immediately become Public Enemy Number One. I was conflicted. I felt ganged up on and knew that this conversation wasn't going to go well if I tried to defy Ethan's desire for soda. Luckily my mom happened to walk in at just the right moment, as Ethan was getting ready to make his demand a little more known.

She tried turning the situation with diet soda. I knew it wouldn't be any better if the soda was diet, but I stayed quiet. As much as it killed me to watch Ethan walk away with his half glass of diet soda, I probably would've done the same thing. It was very upsetting and discouraging.

I had been critical of my mother when it came to Ethan's dietary needs and what seemed like her lack of control over the matter. But at that moment I really began to feel bad for putting so much pressure on her. When you have what feels like the world against you, how are you supposed to stay strong? How do you keep fighting when it feels like you're hitting a brick wall? I mean, there were two of us there on the same side, and Ethan still walked away with his soda. But I knew how it would go if we didn't give in to him. He would've thrown a tantrum, and then it wouldn't just be my uncle giving us dirty looks, it would be at least half of the other people there. This is exactly why I didn't want to be there in the first place. It wasn't a controlled environment. With autism, you need a very controlled environment. You need an escape route, a quiet room, and a bag of tricks to save the day. There was no quiet room, or bag of tricks, and my only escape route seemed to be a bottle of whiskey staring right at me.

As the night continued, I became exactly what I had spoken so critically of: a family member who turned the other cheek and pretended not to see Ethan eat candy or have more soda.I had had my nose in the air, acting like my mother's job wasn't that difficult, that all she had to do was be stricter, when in reality, being stricter would have had my relatives nailing her to the cross.

Inevitably, as Ethan began having more sugar (and Lord knows what else), he got more hyper and giddy. Combine this with the fact that everyone in my family has a stupid, little dog and likes to bring them to family gatherings and the result was a disaster waiting to happen. Ethan wanted to play with them and pinch their stupid, wet, little noses. And like the entitled little bitches they are, those dogs acted like they were too damn good for Ethan. Of course, this only excited him more and more.

My grandpa's sister, Geraldine (or as we called her, Aunt Gerald), has four of those little dogs. She calls them quadruplets and dresses them up in little sweaters and gives them little blankets as they take up space on the couch. She even has a pouch she straps around her waist to carry them in. It's silly. They're stupid, little dogs. They don't need blankets or sweaters. What they need is to be outside, especially if they don't want Ethan pinching their noses. Well, as you may expect, all night long Ethan followed the dogs around wanting to play, and all night long, the damn little rats barked like crazy every time he came near them.

"Oh no, don't let Deets near Princess. Princess bites," Gerald warned. Yeah, well, so do I.I tried my best to keep an eye on Ethan and get the dogs away from him by lightly kicking them until they were out of the room. To keep them off the seats, I put their lounging blankets into a gift bag addressed to Gerald from one of her sisters.

I then became distracted by my cousin Jennifer, who was pushing thirty and seemed to be having a midlife crisis that she thought some whiskey and a little talk with Zack would help fix. I was fully sober and slightly enjoying this conversation when I noticed that Ethan was crying. I excused myself and walked over to him to see what was the matter. Apparently, someone (nobody wanted to mention who) had yelled at Ethan for God knows what. Someone was always yelling at Ethan for something, usually when my mom and I weren't around. At this point, I was ready to snap at somebody. I don't give a shit if someone doesn't like Ethan's behavior or doesn't agree with how he's disciplined. I won't let anyone, under *any* circumstances, scold him, especially those who don't understand Ethan. I don't know who it was or what they told him, but he was surely shaken up. I'll tell you right now, that didn't sit well with me. I'm still his big brother, and as a big brother should, I was ready to kick some ass to protect him. Nobody ended up coming forward, so there was no one to confront, and I ended up just letting my mother know I was ready to go. I was no longer in the mood to continue participating in the evening's festivities.

Shortly after, we went home. At least I walked away with a flask and a bottle of brandy from the White Elephant game, and Mom ended up with a bottle of tequila and a doll, but we won't talk about the doll. I mean, it looked like it had gotten an eye transplant and a bad haircut. That's the thing with the White Elephant game: you either luck out and get something good or you end up with a shitty doll with mix-and-match eyes.

I woke up the next morning, trying to recover from my sugar hangover while I got ready for Christmas part two. We were supposed to go over to my mother's mom's. I was a little more enthusiastic about going to this one.

"Let's go, let's go, let's go. We're going to be late. Come on, let's get ready." I started rushing everyone, figuring that if I didn't, we probably wouldn't get there until New Year's Eve. But at least with my mom's spontaneous baking, we'd be fully stocked with cake.

All in all, the holidays were quite nice. I was actually able to relax and have quality family time, despite the havoc of Christmas Eve. It taught me that I needed to be more present in my time with my family. It also taught me that I seriously needed to cut my mother some slack and help her out more. I also needed to get my stepfather on track. Mom had boarded Ethan's recovery train, but Jeff was still one foot in, one foot out. It was time for me to push his ass on board and keep driving.

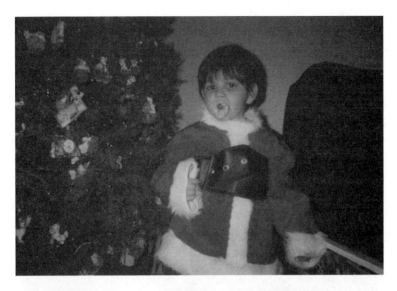

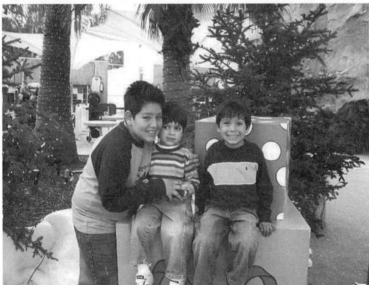

Merry Christmas!

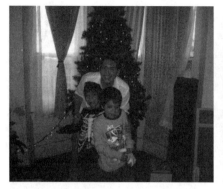

Christmas 2009.

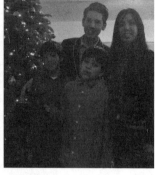

Christmas 2012.

A Shot of Hope

Never judge someone without fully understanding their circumstances, unless they're wearing a pouch to carry their puppies.

CHAPTER TWELVE

The Fight, the Struggle—Now Where's the Triumph?

I've fought. I've struggled. I've wondered, *Where the hell is my triumph?*

This struggle with Ethan (and life in general) has been just that: a *struggle*. I know that there really is no action plan that is guaranteed to work when it comes to autism recovery (or life, for that matter). Yes, there are many therapies and treatments, but the autism spectrum is so diverse that not every child responds the same way. Accepting that is tough.

It's constant trial and error, and sometimes you don't see re-sults as quickly as you'd like. I have often forgotten the *con-stant trial and error* part. It is a continuous journey with no breaks. And with that journey, you have to accept the process, no matter how difficult it may be at times.

At work, my office mate Sarah has a young daughter on the spectrum. Sarah is one of the most educated mommy warriors I know. I often go to her for advice and guidance, both with au-tism and my own personal life. When she brings her daughter into the office, little Caroline runs up to me and says, "Hi, Zack." As much as this lights up my face, it can be a little tough for me to handle. Why can't Ethan run up to me every time he sees me with just as much joy and life in his eyes? Or when Sarah shares a story about something funny Caroline did or said, I'm not gonna lie, it stings a little. I'm not saying I'm jealous of Sarah and Caroline's progress, but . . . okay, maybe I'm a little jealous. Or maybe jealous is the wrong word because I really am so proud of Sarah's progress with Caroline. Maybe I'm just a little disappointed that Ethan isn't at that point yet. Autism is just so unpredictable that there never is a 100 percent guaran-tee that you're going to see the same results as someone else, or any results at all at times. But that's no reason to give up hope.

"I feel guilty," I confessed to my friend Calvin one day.

"What do you feel guilty about?"

I really had to think about it. I knew there was this deep feeling of guilt inside me, but I didn't fully understand where it was coming from. So before I answered him, I asked myself,

What do I feel guilty about? My life isn't terrible. Profession-ally, things are looking up, and personally, I'm a little more put together, at least compared to a couple of years ago. So why feel guilty? And that's when it hit me. I was feeling guilty *because* things were starting to work out for me. And it was all in the midst of Ethan's regression. It didn't feel fair for me to live my own life while he couldn't live his.

Yes, my mom and I had applied biomed and, yes, we saw great results, but after I moved away, it all started to diminish. My mother didn't have her go-to sidekick there as often, and the struggle with the rest of my family wasn't easy for her to fight on her own. I knew leaving was a good step for me to take. It really paid off, but at what expense? At Ethan's?

"I blame myself for Ethan's regression," I told Calvin.

"Is that fair? Is it really your fault?" he replied, sounding a little more empathetic than before.

"Well, if I were around more often, maybe he would be in a better place? Maybe if I weren't so focused on building a career for myself, I could put more time into helping him." Then I stopped myself. Was this realistic? Could I really have put my life on hold to dedicate all of my time to Ethan? Sure, I *could have*, but I still needed to take care of *me*. I didn't have anybody to look after me. As it was, I was in debt at seventeen, crying on my bedroom floor over the financial mess I had made for my-self, thinking of how I was going to get myself out of it. Maybe I put a lot of pressure on myself, but I surely didn't feel like I had either of my parents to take care of me. So, essentially, I *had* to build my own career. I had to go through my own personal struggle to make something of myself. Yes, I did have to take some time to focus on myself. I think I just assumed (or at least hoped) that while I took care of myself, everyone else would take care of Ethan's needs.

We had put a lot of time into Ethan's recovery, but without consistency, recovery is inconsistent. It's like a garden. If you don't maintain it, the plants will slowly start to fail. Autism recovery takes work, time, and a hell of a lot of energy. And it can't all be done by one person. It has to be a team effort. That team is the family.

Sure, Ethan isn't fully recovered right now. We are still going through our process, our own journey. I'll be honest with you about that. But it's not because biomedical treatment doesn't work. This fight with my family has been a rough one. It's hard getting and keeping them focused on it. Biomed isn't easy. That's the harsh reality. It takes a lot of time and dedication and patience. It's a struggle. And sometimes the triumph doesn't come right away. That takes time too.

One thing I learned I needed to do was appreciate everything I, myself, have been through, and everything my family has been through. Sometimes I just want to give up. I look at what appears to be a long road ahead without taking the time to look back and really appreciate how far we've all come, how much stronger we've all become. I've been pushed to limits I never imagined I would reach.

In the midst of trying to deal with Ethan's regression and my own sibling guilt, the shit hit the fan in my personal life.

Things got messy. I was juggling life as a young adult in college. I was working a part-time job, writing books, doing stand-up and motivational speaking tours, organizing and hosting charity events, and producing a weekly show. In the midst of all this, I got my heart broken. Badly. But at least I found out that I had one (always look at the positive, right?).

Life doesn't always give you what you want, at least not *when* you want it. It gives it to you when you're ready for it. Life isn't a magic lamp with a genie who will grant you anything you want before your very eyes. Nothing worth obtaining is easy. You want the triumph? You have to get dirty and do the work. If Zoila wants her paycheck at the end of the week, she has to mop those floors and clean them dishes. That money isn't going to flow right in. Zoila has to put in the work. We all do.

No, I'll be honest. I don't have all the answers. I don't think anybody ever does or ever should. Life is about evolving into more mature versions of ourselves. With each stage, there are new lessons to be learned. Whether it's learning how to ride a bike, learning how to write an essay, learning how to have sex, learning how to make a marriage work, or learning how to drink a glass of orange juice without having your dentures fall out, life's a series of lessons. So don't be stubborn. Allow yourself to actually learn them and appreciate the process. Then, one day, probably when you least expect it, *bam!* The triumph will come!

A Shot of Hope
If you didn't take anything away from this chapter, reread it.

CHAPTER THIRTEEN

Insanity Ensues

Following the holidays, I knew it was time to start implementing a plan. I wanted Ethan to begin seeing a treatment physician, someone who had lots of experience in treating autism. He had seen one back in 2010, but it was just a brief consultation, and the conclusion was that he had too much yeast in his system. We were supposed to go back for a follow-up, but things didn't end up working out. Thus, Ethan's regression.

Mom had expressed to me that Ethan was having major problems with insomnia. "He won't sleep. At all. He keeps us up all night. I literally had to beg Jeff the other night to pick him up because I was so tired and needed to get some sleep."

I suggested giving him some melatonin, but she said that wasn't working.

The following week I was working with Dr. Jerry Kartzinel on a live Q&A session. He and I had met a few years back when I interviewed him for a web series I was hosting. One of the questions Dr. Jerry got was regarding sleep. In his answer, he mentioned that sleep problems could be related to constipation, among other things. Later that day I asked my mom if she thought Ethan may be constipated or had some sort of digestive problem.

"Yes!" she said, and mentioned how bloated he would get at times. EJ had had a number of digestive issues since he was a baby, as did I, so I knew it was practically inevitable for Ethan to follow in our same tummy-aching footsteps. Who knew it wasn't normal to go to the bathroom only once a week? As it was, anytime my stomach hurt, my grandma just told me that meant I had to use the bathroom. Little did we know it was due to food intolerances and constipation.

I mentioned to my co-worker Sarah that I was looking to find a treatment doctor for Ethan. She mentioned how great Dr. Jerry was. After all, he did write *Healing and Preventing Autism*. Though I had known him for years, I'd never thought to ask if he'd take Ethan on as a patient. If I could pick any doctor, it would be Dr. Jerry. I've had the privilege of interviewing him, working alongside him, and I loved his book. The way he describes autism is just so on-point: "Autism is an abnormal response to everyday stimuli." He doesn't talk about autism in a bad way, but simply that children with autism normally have a common list of comorbid conditions that are medically treatable. When those conditions are treated, the overall autism improves. He describes it so well and in a way that's easy to understand. That's why I love his website. It's got everything you need to know in clear, easy-to-grasp posts.

I put in a call to his office to see if he had the availability to take on another patient—my brother, to be specific. A few days later I heard back.

"Oh my God," I said, spitting out my coffee. "Oh my God," I repeated as I turned to Sarah.

"What now?" she asked. "Another self-proclaimed swamp witch on Twitter attacking you?"

"No, Dr. Jerry's agreed to take Ethan on as a patient!"

"What? That's fantastic, Zack!"

I was honestly overwhelmed. I could not believe it. I wanted to cry. My dying hope was being reignited. It was another step closer to Ethan's recovery. I literally had to get up, leave the room, and take a moment. I walked over to the restroom and just stood over the sink with my head down. I looked up. "Thank You," I prayed. "Just . . . Thank You," I said to God.

I had done a lot of crazy stuff, made many crazy comments, and even hit a lot of lows over the years. But somehow, for some reason, despite the loads of "crazy" karma I believed I deserved, things were working out. All of the hard work over the years was now paying off. Sometimes I really didn't think it would. I never thought my family would have this opportunity. There were so many nights I thought it was never going to happen, that one day Ethan might have to be dependent on one of us and might never have the ability to live on his own, or have his own job, or marry someone he really loves. I know I had told people over the years that there's no such thing as false hope, but sometimes I really felt my hope slipping. Things just didn't look good before, but now they were looking pretty damn great. And it didn't hurt that I was in the restroom that had my favorite mirror in it. I looked hella sexy as usual, but this time when I looked into the mirror I saw a kid working hard to make his family proud. I saw a brother working at giving his little brother the best he could possibly give him despite all the criticism, all the trolls, all the teary nights. I saw a real person with strength and courage. And I saw myself actually believing that one day I would have a real conversation with my brother. I saw real hope.

I walked back to my desk and texted my mom, "See you for dinner at 7? I have huge news." Later that night, I met with her and Ethan for our usual weekly dinner. I told her about Dr. Jerry and that I had already booked our first appointment. She was excited. I told her we had a little paperwork to send back to his office, but that this was all real. We were finally making some real progress.

As she and I began filling out some of the information for Dr. Jerry's office, we went over Ethan's history. She told me that she had consumed large amounts of tuna fish while pregnant with Ethan. She brought up again that his "light switch" seemed to flick off after his eight-month shots. She also brought up the silver fillings he had put in his mouth around the time he turned four. Reflecting on all of this, I began to realize that

Ethan was clearly suffering some heavy-metal poisoning. With the fish and the metals in the vaccinations and the silver fillings, things were beginning to make a lot more sense. I had never really known about Mom's fish binge during her pregnancy, nor did I even remember Ethan's silver fillings. I mean, I remember when he had them put in and how concerned Mom was at the time, but during his recovery, I had failed to connect with the other components.

I went home and looked into mercury and heavy-metal toxicity. I was mortified at how many symptoms matched up with Ethan's and how many symptoms also coincided with "symptoms of autism."

It's one thing to know your brother has autism. It's another thing to see everything right in front of you that clearly displays your brother was poisoned by the food purchased at the supermarket, and by the doctor and dentist entrusted with his health. It was sickening to me. Sure, the thimerosal in the vaccine is only in "trace amounts." Sure, the mercury in fish is *very little*. Sure, the metal in silver fillings isn't enough to cause harm to that extent. Sure, but what about the combination of all of them? What then? That's the part that troubles me. As someone who watched his brother's regression unfold, it left an ugly feeling in the pit of my stomach to see that this is the reality of the world that we live in. But I was determined to focus on getting Ethan better and improving his autism. Now that we knew metal toxicity was clearly something that we needed to address, I knew that it would help us take the next step in the right direction.

"It just blows my mind," I told Sarah.

"I know," she agreed, as I shared what I had discovered about Ethan and what clearly looked like an adverse reaction to heavy metals.

"So, I think when we see Dr. Jerry, that's something we're really going to want to address. But just think of how much better he's done while on GF/CF, and now how much more he's likely to improve with detox."

Initially, I was worried. Yes, I knew that he needed to be detoxed and he needed to get the metals out of his body. That was crucial, but I had heard all of the controversy that came with chelation therapy, which is basically the removal of heavy metals from the body. Most of the controversy came from mainstream media outlets that often profiled treatments inaccurately or with a particular bias. I kept an open mind and decided to see what Dr. Jerry had to say, but the appointment was still a few weeks away and I had a million other things to still take care of in the meantime. So I filed it away for the moment.

That same week, I had a call with a producer I had worked with on a couple of projects. She had done some amazing work and I was really impressed with her skills in film. We had chatted a couple of months back about potentially doing a public service announcement to raise awareness for autism, which eventually became an idea to film a documentary about autism.

After bouncing around ideas and sitting on this one for a bit, she came back to me and told me her production company was interested in producing the documentary and that they wanted to make me the primary focus.

"I just find you to be a very interesting person," she told me. Flattered, I agreed. The documentary was going to follow my life trying to help Ethan while juggling all the other projects I was working on. I've always been candid and I thought this would be a great way to show people what a family really goes through when autism is brought into the mix. I also thought this would be a great opportunity to really make Ethan's recovery a main focus for everyone. If his progress was going to be documented, everyone in my family would have to be on board 100 percent so that there was actual progress to document. There was really no excuse at this point. Naturally, like being on a diet, you're more likely to "cheat" if nobody's around. But if there's a camera on you, there's really no room to "cheat."

"I want to make it clear that you have full access to me and my life and you can pry into every single bit of it that you want. However, I want to be clear that when it comes to my family, and primarily with my mom and brothers, there are boundaries," I told the producer before even looking at the agreement. I was totally game for this. It would draw attention to autism, recovery, and treatment options. But I wanted to make sure that my mother's household and my brothers' lives were not invaded in any way. People may see me as a little territorial, but I think I'm just very protective of the things and the people who are the most important to me. I just know how cruel this world can be and putting my brother on that platform was something I held very strong reservations against. I made sure to run the idea by my mother first, and then, if she agreed, we would move forward. We decided to title the project *Sibling*

Warrior: Healing My Brother's Autism and expected to begin filming the following month.

In addition to refocusing my attention on Ethan's recovery, and now signing up to do a documentary, my part-time office job was getting more demanding. And just when I thought I couldn't take on any more, I got a text message from the lovely Ashlee Holmes. Ashlee was one of the original cast members from Bravo's *Real Housewives of New Jersey* and was also a big advocate for autism.

Ashlee and I had met when we hosted the first Rock Now for Autism benefit concert I had put together the year before. She, like me, has a young brother with autism and was living in Los Angeles at the time. I thought she would be a great fit to host this event with me. I reached out to her on Twitter and confirmed with her one week before the event. We met, literally, twenty-four hours before the event. Luckily, we had instant chemistry and clicked. I was so glad, especially since I was extremely stressed out. This event was by far one of the most difficult events I have ever had to organize, which is why with everything on my plate, I was certain I could not do another one, at least not anytime soon. Or, at least not until Ashlee texted me.

"So, I have tons of friends interested in being a part of this year's event," Ashlee texted.

Shit, I thought. Rock Now had been so far from my radar that I didn't even know how to reply. I love Ashlee. She's amazing and has electric energy. There was no way I could tell her I didn't want to do another event. So I entertained the idea for a bit and somehow during that texting conversation, we picked a date, and Ashlee announced it on Instagram.

"You know I'm crazy, right?" I texted Sarah.

"What did you do now?" she replied.

"So, Rock Now is happening this May. Ashlee and I have already begun planning."

"Well, that's so you. Go big or go home!"

Sarah was right. Go big or go home, roll into a ball, pull a sheet over my head, and never come back out. I have a tendency of overcommitting myself at times, or a lot more often than is probably healthy for my sanity and blood pressure. I'm learning. It's a lesson I continue to learn (and continue to forget). It's usually not until about the eighth time around that I actually learn the lesson. But I promise, by the ninth time, I've got that shit down!

A Shot of Hope

Don't overcommit yourself or you'll likely end up in the loony bin. I'm already packing my bags!

CHAPTER FOURTEEN

All in a Day's Work

On the day of Ethan's appointment with Dr. Jerry, I popped out of bed ready to go. I had just downloaded a new sleep app on my phone with an amazing morning alarm. Instead of the typical buzzers, this one plays very soft, soothing music as it gradually works the waves in your brain and tells you to wake up.

I definitely need to get this app for Ethan, I thought.

Things were going great, despite how high my level of stress had been lately. Between everything I was juggling and the latest season of ABC's *Scandal* coming to an end, I thought I was going to have a heart attack. But surprisingly, things were starting to look up. Then I began scrolling through my phone . . .

It had been almost two months since I had booked Ethan's appointment with Dr. Jerry, signed on to do the documentary, and agreed to host another Rock Now. Things were moving along. Filming had officially begun, we had a venue for Rock Now, and our talent lineup was in the process of being finalized. I had been organizing events for almost six years now, so I had most of my ducks in a row and was kicking ass. Ticket sales were just about to officially go on sale when I got a text message from Ashlee. She was unfortunately having to back out of the Rock Now benefit event we were planning together and unexpectedly head back to New Jersey.

I took a very, very deep breath. This event was undoubtedly on my top-three list for why my blood pressure had been skyrocketing all month. I took another deep breath. "I'm not going to let this ruin my day," I reassured myself. "Everything will be okay."

We had scheduled Ethan's appointment with Dr. Jerry to be part of the documentary, so it was going to be a big day and I wasn't going to let a little bump in the road throw me off, even though losing your co-council and co-host for your big annual benefit concert is arguably more than just a little bump in the road. I just hoped that my mother would arrive on time.

"Be here tomorrow at *nine*," I told her the day before, with an extra emphasis on the *nine*.

Our appointment was at 10:00 A.M. and it would be a long drive from Los Angeles to Irvine.

"*Nine*, Mother," I repeated.

"Okay, I'll be there at *nine* tomorrow," she promised.

While I waited for her, I drank a tall glass of water to wake up my digestive system and then began brewing some coffee. I walked over and flipped on the TV and began watching a little bit of *Charmed*. It brought back nostalgia from when I was a kid and used to watch it with a gallon of ice cream every Thursday night on the WB. I needed something to calm me down.

I then hopped in the shower and began getting ready. I wasn't in much of a rush because I was preparing myself to kill extra time in case my mother didn't arrive promptly at 9:00 A.M.

To my pleasant surprise, she pulled up right in front of the house at exactly 9:01 A.M. Right on time. I was very impressed. *Maybe this day won't be so bad after all*, I thought. I was really excited. *Really* excited. This was our first big appointment and it was going to play a crucial part in the documentary we had been filming. I couldn't believe this was becoming real.

I hurried out to the car to meet Mom and Ethan and head on our way. I pulled up the GPS on my phone and the time estimate showed an exact one-hour arrival time. I could live with that. Arriving exactly at 10:00 A.M. wouldn't be a bad thing. We would still technically be on time.

What I didn't factor in, however, was Siri acting up, missing our freeway exits, and the constant phone calls on the way over, which then also interfered with the GPS. Luckily, two of the calls were from an amazingly supportive friend who was helping me pull in sponsors for Rock Now with news that she was close to sealing the deal and would have confirmation by the following week. I felt confident, but I never like to celebrate until the check is in the bank. You'd be surprised how many people like to cancel at the last minute.

The next call that came was from the executive producer of our documentary.

"Hello," I answered, assuming that she was calling to tell me that they had just arrived at the Kartzinel Wellness Center and were setting up to film.

"Hey, Zack. Quick question: If we're trying to get there on the 210 freeway, where would we exit?"

Now, getting from Pasadena (where she was coming from) to Irvine isn't easy, I'll admit that. There are more curves and turns on the way over than on a Kardashian's body. You have to switch from one freeway to the next and then merge onto another . . . It's complicated. But the 210 freeway was still about forty minutes away from where we were. It takes you in a completely different direction.

"I'm not sure. We took the 10 to the 57. And then somehow we're going to get to the 5 and exit there."

"Oh. Okay. Actually, I think we're almost there."

"Oh . . . Okay, then. See you in a bit," I said as I hung up the phone.

"What'd they say?" my mom asked.

"That they're not going to be there before us."

I looked at the estimated arrival time: 10:20 A.M. I then emailed Dr. Jerry's office and told them we were running slightly behind schedule, but would be there soon.

We made it right around our estimate, but wanted to kill some time for the crew to arrive, so we decided to stop by

Starbucks. I knew it was extremely rude, but if we had to sit for forty minutes and wait for the crew to arrive, I knew Ethan would get antsy and begin acting up, especially since he'd been sitting in a car for over an hour.

Then I got an email back from Dr's Jerry's office.

"Hey, Zack, what's your status? Dr. Jerry and I have a business meeting at eleven we can't miss."

"Shit," I muttered. I then hopped on the phone to call the crew for a status update. They were still at least half an hour away and by this time it was already 10:40 A.M.

"I am so pissed right now," I told my mom. "What the hell am I working so damn hard for? Shit needs to get done, and I'm the one doing it and nobody else seems to be picking up any of the slack."

She didn't say anything. Between Ashlee canceling, the crew running behind, and my frustration over getting everyone on track for Ethan, I was ready to explode. My tolerance level was just reaching its boiling point.

We then arrived at the Kartzinel Wellness Center, and I ran in to find David sitting at the front desk. David is Dr. Jerry's son, who had been emailing with me back and forth since we first booked the appointment. He's incredibly kind, and I felt horrible that not only did we make them wait, but now they had a meeting to jump into.

"I am *so* sorry, David," I began apologizing.

"Look, Zack. Don't worry about it. I understand. Traffic is tough. You can never predict it."

"I know," I said, feeling even guiltier since we were actually just five minutes away grabbing a Starbucks, trying to kill time for our crew. It was a detour that had cost us time with people who have been very kind to my family.

Not only were we not going to be able to film with Dr. Jerry that day, but we weren't going to have time for an appointment at all. The visit that I had been looking forward to for weeks was now out the window. And I was beginning to see my sanity go along with it.

"We're going to have to reschedule," David told me. The next available date was a month and a half later.

"Okay," I said. I was upset because the majority of filming was to take place in the next two months, and my manuscript was due before then. I really wanted to cover our appointment with Dr. Jerry and the protocols we implemented following his advice. But at this point, it was just out of the question.

I gave David a list of the supplements I had ordered for Ethan and everything else we were looking to try. I asked him to run it by Dr. Jerry and at least give us a little direction, if possible. The only challenge is that every child is different, and without proper examination, there's not much that can be done. Dr. Jerry reviewed the list and came out to speak with me for a minute before he had to run off to his meeting. David then addressed a few other questions we had. I was so appreciative of the time he took away from participating in the meeting to help us out. The crew arrived just in time to catch a little footage.

We then left the office and my mother began rushing back to LA because she planned to go back to work. She's a school bus driver. So she picks the kids up and takes them to school, works in the office during the school day, and then drives them home. It was a half day at school and she wanted to make it back in time. I had never in my life seen her drive so fast. I then thought back to a number of other times her speed-racer skills would have come in handy and were very absent. I then made a mental note for future reference.

"Well, at least we got some stuff filmed," I told her as I shrugged my shoulders. I was really bummed not so much about the filming, but that we were now going to be delayed in everything else pertaining to Ethan's recovery. I don't like delays. You should see me when my flight's delayed at the airport. I turn into a cast member from the *Real Housewives of Atlanta*.

My mother dropped me back at home and rushed to work. My younger brother Shawn (from one of my father's previous relationships after my mother) had been staying over recently and wanted to go to the mall to buy a new pair of shoes. I knew it would probably be dangerous, since I didn't have extra money. That month I happened to be trying out the Paleo diet, so all of the organic foods I had been substituting for my regular dishes were weighing heavily on my wallet. Not to mention the nontoxic mattress I had just purchased my aunt for my new baby cousin, and then the supplements I bought for me and Ethan at Dr. Jerry's office. My finances were really starting to run thin. But I just needed to be anywhere but home, so I agreed to go to the mall with him.

As Shawn and I walked through the mall, I got a phone call from the management team of one of the musicians I was looking to book for Rock Now. He was a friend of Ashlee's so I assumed he would do the event pro bono. His management team wasn't interested in booking a pro bono gig and were trying to get us to pay a thousand dollars for a fifteen-minute set, which they claimed was "*significantly lower* than the standard quote." I didn't really give a shit. It was *significantly higher* than we could afford to pay for a charity event for a 501(c)(3) nonprofit organization that helps kids. Let's just say that the conversation didn't go well.

"I'm not even going to ask," Shawn said, and kept walking.

After arriving home later that night, I realized, yes, it had been a pretty shitty day. But despite how much seemed to have gone wrong, I didn't really have the chance to let any of my current projects slip. Ethan still needed assistance, and I still had to move forward with Rock Now, with or without Ashlee. And clearly without a certain musician who will remain nameless.

I got a couple of questions in to the doctor and his office, which were addressed, and did some more research on my own. Ethan needed to be on a very strict GF/CF diet with very little sugar intake. I actually convinced my mother to get him to try the Paleo diet. Actually, it was *her* idea. He needed a good multivitamin, which I got from Dr. Jerry. He needed omega-3s, probiotics, antifungals, antivirals, digestive enzymes, and something to help kick some yeast ass. He also needed to start detoxing, and we needed to get my mother's house detoxified. You'd be surprised how toxic your household cleaning products and furniture are.

I hopped on the phone and chatted with company reps. I sent emails back and forth with questions. I was determined. This was it. Screw how crappy one day was. I was not going to let it knock us off our game.

One thing David reminded me when I was asking him questions at Dr. Jerry's office was that not every child responds the same way. Some kids respond really well to certain products and others might not respond as strongly, if at all. It's why trial and error is important, but it's also why it's important to not cry "cure" when something does work. A lot of people do see great results, but it's still not a good idea to shout this from the rooftops because what works for your kid may not work for every child. Every child is unique and has his own needs, which is exactly what I needed to remember with Ethan.

A Shot of Hope
A bad day doesn't mean you have a bad life. It just means you need a really strong drink.

CHAPTER FIFTEEN

Progress, At Last!

"I just don't know what to do," my mom told me. "It's just who they are and I can't change them." The "they" she was referring to was my grandparents.

"Well, you know I'm here for you."

We had just finished filming for the day for our documentary, *Sibling Warrior*. I had ordered Ethan an infrared sauna, and it had been delivered earlier that day, so I had come over to help set it up. It was much more complicated than it looked. I assumed you just put the four walls together on top of the base and then covered it with the ceiling. Boy, was I wrong.

Yes, there were four walls, a base, and a ceiling, but everything was heavy, everything needed assembling, and then there were a bunch of wires to be connected. I tried as best as I could to help put it together, but I wasn't of much help, not that I really ever am when it comes to manual labor.

I had heard that infrared saunas were helpful for kids with autism but had never really understood why. It was all about the detox. But I never understood what kind of detox these kids needed and how a sauna would actually benefit them.

I ended up reaching out to Sunlighten, which is a company specializing in quality infrared saunas. They supported the cause, so I figured they knew a lot about the benefits of saunas for people with autism. We decided it would be best to get Ethan a two-person sauna. Sunlighten also carried an individual sauna that looked like a sleeping bag, but just looking at it made me anxious, and I decided it might not be the best choice for Ethan either. Besides, the two-person sauna would allow someone to join him.

A couple of weeks later, I surprised my mom at dinner and told her it would be my gift to them for their birthdays. I would've gotten the sauna regardless, but since I had forgotten to buy her a gift, I figured a signature two-person sauna would do the trick. And it did. She was over the moon.

I explained to her that the sauna was designed to help Ethan's detoxification of heavy metals out of his system, as well as everyday toxins, like pesticides. It would also help boost his immunity and calm him down, which would be helpful before bed. We checked it first with Dr. Jerry, and he assured us that our bodies' best way of getting rid of toxins is through sweating.

I had used an infrared sauna for a few months before getting one for Ethan and loved the benefits, which is why I was so intrigued to learn more about them and eventually got Ethan to start using one.

After we assembled it, we showed it to Ethan and he got really excited. It was a giant wooden box just for him with all sorts of fancy buttons and music. What kid wouldn't love getting a surprise larger than himself, regardless of what it was?

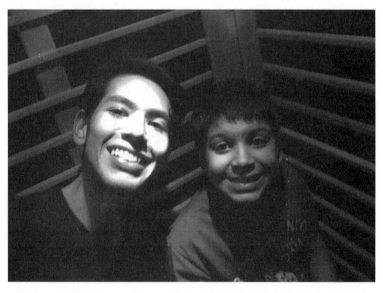

Sauna time!

After two hours of assembling, my mom and I (along with our cameraman for the day) went to the kitchen to go over our plan of action with Ethan. I pulled out all his supplements and started talking to her about what we should try out and for how long. She seemed a little tired and not really in the mood to have this conversation. I wasn't sure if this was because we were on camera and she was a little uncomfortable, or if she was really tired and really not in the mood. The excitement of the sauna had worn off, and she seemed a little down about something.

I continued to blaze through my tutorial of how to implement everything and when to start trying what. I even let her know what to expect from which supplements. After dinner, we wrapped up filming and began settling down for the day. She was giving me a ride home since I took the train to meet her. Again, in the car, I reminded her of the importance of consistency in giving Ethan these supplements, using the sauna, and, most of all, maintaining his diet. We were going to begin a yeast cleanse and needed to ensure that he wasn't feeding the yeast by consuming too much sugar. Giving him too much juice to drink or too many carbs to eat would just counteract the cleanse, so his diet needed to be as clean as possible.

"It's very important that you stay on top of this," I reminded her.

"I know," she kept assuring me.

I was worried. We had tried several times to get Ethan on track but kept hitting a number of road bumps. But I was going to make sure this time things would be different. No more half-assed shit. It was time to make it happen.

Ethan was still having major behavioral issues and he wasn't very verbal. At least not to the degree he should've been.

He also wasn't social at all. This really disappointed me. I wanted him to have friends and play with other kids his own age. He was still off in his own world. I wanted to tackle each of these obstacles and hopefully really provide him with some clarity.

That's when my mother started really opening up to me. She went on about how difficult it was for her to keep Ethan on the diet, especially since he would go to my grandmother's house after school until my mom got out of work. My grandparents were still very much against the diet, using the same excuses they did seven years ago. It was the same damn conversation every time. I felt like I was working with Lindsay Lohan. No matter how many rehab attempts, it always ended up the same way.

"It just pisses me off," I told her.

"I'm thinking of just leaving work," she replied. "I mean, how else can I make sure he's eating right unless I'm with him all day? They're just not willing to change, no matter how hard I try to work with them. I've tried fighting with them. I've tried begging for their help. They just will not change." She was running out of options. There really wasn't anyone who was available and trustworthy enough to babysit him, and paying for additional childcare just wasn't in the budget.

I continued to reassure her that I was there for her. Seeing her this defeated made me feel angry and hurt. I knew how my grandparents were. They would never mean to hurt Ethan or not help him; it was just that they could not wrap their heads around the fact that Ethan could not eat certain foods and that he would really benefit from not eating those foods. Shit, we could all benefit from not eating those foods. They kept on with the whole "diet" thing. "Kids shouldn't be on diets." It was the same conversation over and over. It was exhausting.

The next week I had a call with one of the head producers for *Sibling Warrior*. "I know it's a conversation I need to have with them. I'm just worried. And I'm worried about having it on camera and how they might respond," I told the producer about confronting my grandparents.

"Yeah, I get that," she replied.

I knew it was a crucial part of the documentary to show this aspect of our struggle, but at the same time, I didn't want to blindside my family with this. I also didn't want them to be portrayed in a negative light. But yet, at the same time, here was my mother considering leaving her job to stay at home full-time to care for Ethan. I was stuck between a rock and a hard place.

I hoped getting this conflict on film might help my family give the diet a little more consideration. But I also knew that it could backfire and that they might shut down or retaliate. That's the thing with documentaries: they portray only what's in a set time frame, never the picture in its entirety. I knew I would never hear the end of it if my family was portrayed negatively and I had done nothing to stop it. My grandparents and uncle are not bad people. It's just been so hard that their actions have worked against what my mom and I have tried to achieve for Ethan.

I kept debating whether I wanted to address the issue with them on camera, hoping to find "the right time" to do it. If it happened on camera, great. If it didn't, then it didn't. Eventually, it did happen. After hearing more stories from my mom, my brother EJ, and my aunt about Ethan being given food he couldn't have, I decided it was best to gently address the issue with my grandma.

I explained to her the difficulty of the circumstances and my frustrations with my mom likely not being fully on board. I knew if I put the blame elsewhere it might get her to be more attentive. I also explained how expensive it was becoming for me with Ethan's doctor bills, lab testing, and vitamins and supplements, as I wanted to help take care of that to lessen the burden on my mother. I knew if I could get some sympathy from her by explaining how much it was not just affecting Ethan, but now me too, she would be more likely to jump on board with us, seeing the chain reaction of her defiance. She went on to tell me that she had been trying, but I knew she could likely make a little more of an effort.

"I know it's not easy. But if we just all do our part with him when he's with each of us, at the end of the day, we can at least say we did all that we could," I told her. And she agreed to. It went a lot smoother than I was expecting. I walked out praising Jesus for the ease of what could've been a heated conversation of banter and blame.

A couple of weeks later, I was heading back to my mom's house to help her put in Ethan's new bed. I had ordered him a special intelliBED, which is a nontoxic mattress made with organic cotton that would help reduce his exposure to toxins. I was shocked to find out how many chemicals are in the average bed! Everything's sprayed with flame retardants, which then off-gas while you sleep. That's insane. Ethan already has a hard time detoxing, which is why we got him the sauna. There was really no point to detoxing if he was just going to be taking the toxins right back in.

I made my mother start switching over to nontoxic cleaning products and buying food from local farmer's markets, which I ended up doing too. I got so paranoid after reading about all this crap and off-gassing that I even bought my aunt an intelliBED crib mattress for her new baby girl. The last thing I wanted was another family member with a severe toxic overload. My mother and I are also now currently in the process of buying our own nontoxic mattresses. Now I'm all about nontoxic, super-detox, clean eating.

It's actually kind of sad how excited I get when I find new cleaning products. At twenty-one, my excitement should be in being able to legally drink, not being able to find a fragrance-free multi-surface cleaner.

It reminded me of when I saw a psychic and she told me I was going to live a very long life. At first, it sounded like a real nightmare. When I look at a lot of old people, they don't always look very happy. Most of them don't make aging look fun at all. With the aches and pains, the oxygen tanks, and the bags of medication, becoming an old man was not something on my bucket list. But now that I think about it, with my go-green and clean new lifestyle, I really wouldn't be surprised if I lived until I was two hundred. Just wait, I'll make it there. I suggest you start doing the same if you plan to make it there too.

The day before Ethan's new bed arrived I texted my mom to remind her it was coming.

"Is it a mattress or the whole bed?" she asked.

"The whole thing. Mattress, box spring, bed frame. They're going to set it up on the spot."

"Okay. It's a full, right?"

"Queen."

"Oh okay. I thought a full."

"I asked you five times if you wanted a full or a queen. And you told me every time to get a queen. You never said a full."

"LOL, somewhere in my head I thought I later said full. I guess I never did. I dreamt it."

Ah, Nancy, I thought.

"I guess so. Is the queen going to fit?" I asked her.

"I hope so."

"Well, you better start moving furniture around tonight."

"I am."

Sometimes I wonder if she purposely disregards things, or if she just has a bad memory. I asked her if she needed my help moving anything else out the next morning. The delivery was scheduled for 8:00 A.M. She told me that it'd be helpful if I stopped by, so I agreed to come over early in the morning before I had to head out to class later that day. It was the end of my spring semester, so not only did I have a term paper due that day, but I was also prepping for finals. I was hoping she might not need my help, but she did. And that was fine. I didn't mind. It's not like I was all that excited to run to campus to write a five-page paper.

I met up with my mother the next morning and we went back to her house. "We've got to hurry," I told her. "I just got a text from one of our camera guys. He's there already to film."

"He's there? Already?"

"Yeah."

"Oh man, I didn't even clean. The house is a mess! I haven't been home all weekend."

"Well, it's not like you didn't know we were filming today."

"I know, but I didn't think they'd be here this early."

"And you're wearing a Dodger hoodie? That's pretty gangster."

"I know! How embarrassing," she replied, as we laughed about her thug-life outfit. Her LA roots were really coming out that day.

When we got to the house, we quickly began cleaning while the camera was set up.

Meanwhile, we were trying to get the boys' room squared away. They had bunk beds that we had to take out to make room for Ethan's new bed. They were a little heavy for my fragile self and my tiny mother, but we managed.

"Zack? Doing manual labor?" the cameraman joked. "I'm glad I'm catching this on film."

"Ha, ha. Very funny," I told him. "I know how to make shit happen."

Shortly after that, two delivery men arrived and brought in Ethan's new bed. It was so comfy! It had a layer of intelliGEL that made it feel like I was sleeping in the clouds! It was amazing.

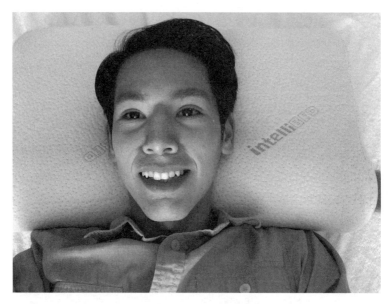

Hijacking Ethan's new bed! Like sleeping on a cloud . . .

I asked my mom how Ethan had been doing lately. "How's he doing with the sauna?"

"Good. At first, the heat was a little tough for him to adjust to, but he's been good."

"That's good."

"Now I just tell him to get ready to do sauna and he'll go grab his things and we'll go right in. So he's gotten used to it. And he's started to sweat more, which is good."

"That *is* good. And how's he doing with the supplements? How's the yeast cleanse going?"

"It's going good."

"Have you seen any difference in him lately?"

"Yes! To the average person, it might not seem that way, but I can definitely see it. It's not major, but it's noticeable. He's calmer. He's more responsive. The other day his therapist came over and was trying to work with him. Ethan told him that his stomach wasn't feeling well and he had a headache, which was really big, because normally he would just hold his head and I'd have to figure out what was the matter. Now he's starting to respond more, so I don't have to figure out what's wrong as much, which is good. He also responds better to discipline."

"That's good!"

"I know. Granted, he would get what he wanted a lot, but now I'm enforcing discipline a lot more, and he's really responding to it. Versus before, I couldn't tell if he just wasn't listening or if there was actually something he wasn't comprehending. So that's gotten better."

"And how's his sleep doing?"

"Mmmm . . ." she said with a squint. "It's better. It's not great, but now I can tell him it's time for bed and he'll start to get ready for bed, whereas before, he wouldn't do that. It was always a fight to get to bed. So he's more responsive in that sense. I think in the past week and a half there have been only two instances where I had trouble getting him to sleep."

"That's really good!"

Then I asked how he was doing with the diet.

"Better," she told me. "When I take him to Grandma's, I'm more strict with them. Every day I tell her what she needs to get him for after school. So I'll tell her to buy some fish and some rice and she's starting to listen, which is a big improvement." That really *was* a big improvement.

"But I'm not going to work this summer," my mom continued. "I'm going to take the summer off to stay home with him and focus on him."

"That's good," I told her. I had no critiques for anything she was doing. She was really stepping up. She went on about all the little improvements Ethan had been making after only two weeks on the new supplements. We had gotten him started on a good multivitamin, had continued his digestive enzymes, and had now been doing a two-week yeast cleanse. The following week we were scheduled to start him on a very good omega-3 supplement.

A Shot of Hope

Sometimes all people need to get them going is a little nudge . . . with a bulldozer.

CHAPTER SIXTEEN

A More Silver Lining

Just a few days after putting in Ethan's new bed, my mom texted me. "Day 3 last night. His sleep has improved. He falls asleep much faster, obeys the rule that the iPad needs to be put away, and hasn't woken up."

"Ah, very cool!" I replied.

She went on to explain how she started implementing a higher dosage of melatonin. She would start with one immediate release capsule to help him fall asleep and one time-release capsule to help him stay asleep throughout the night. "The combo has been the trick. Oh, and he settles down for me to read him a story. This is where he falls asleep right when I start reading," she continued. "As active as he was last night, he dropped after his bath and a story. Again, this consistency is new."

I was over-the-moon excited. The night before, we had met up for our weekly dinner. I was running late after work, so we met up at the local farmer's market. When I got there, Ethan seemed to be very hyper. He kept running off and seemed very excited about something. He was also spinning a lot, which is a common trait of "stimming," a behavioral symptom of autism. I was worried my mother wasn't following up with the protocols we had in place.

We had tried a few times before to get Ethan on track. But things never ended up being followed through. I guess you could say life happens. But this time, I was certain we were going to see progress and we were really going to help Ethan.

After the farmer's market, we had gone to one of my favorite Southern California eateries. It's a cafeteria-style little restaurant called Lemonade. I love it because it is simple, tasty, and they have lots of options that meet our dietary needs. Since I arrived late, everyone had already eaten at the farmer's market. So really, we were just going for me and so my aunt could try the place out. It was her first time joining us for our weekly dinners. I ordered my favorite spicy pineapple chicken and a portion of almond cauliflower with golden raisins. I got some salmon for Mom and Ethan to share and some brisket. It was delicious. We each ordered a different flavor of lemonade. Mom and EJ got cucumber mint, my aunt got blood orange, and I ordered a sugar-free blueberry mint lemonade to share with Ethan. The lemonades were huge, so it was perfect for two.

While eating, Ethan kept blowing bubbles with his lemonade, causing it to splash all over the table. He thought it was the funniest thing. It made a mess. Again, I was worried he might not have been behaving because he wasn't following a proper diet.

"Ethan, that's enough," my mother told him. "Give me your lemonade," she said before taking it away. I was very impressed. She was taking command, and he was listening without throwing a tantrum or screaming. He raised his voice a little, telling her no, but she followed through and he listened.

"If you want it back, you have to ask for it," she told him.

"I want my lemonade," Ethan said.

"Say please."

"I want my lemonade, please."

I couldn't believe it! Normally, he'd say, at the most, three words. And usually they were grumbled. Rarely did he ever say full or complete sentences. Now he had just said a full five-word sentence right in front of me. I was ready to begin shouting, "Hallelujah!" and break out into song.

"Good job, Ethan," I said.

He blew a couple more bubbles before the lemonade was taken away completely, but he was starting to say full sentences. And nobody had to feed him the words. Just last month, when we'd gone out to dinner, I'd asked him, "Do you want lemonade?" He didn't respond.

"Ethan, do you want lemonade?" I asked again with no response. "Ethan? Yes or no?"

"Yes," he said in a very low voice, almost as if he was just repeating me.

"He always says that," EJ piped in. "Ask him yes or no to anything and he'll always just say yes."

So from having to feed him "yes" to having him make a full command sentence was a pretty big deal. And then when my mom began texting me about his improved sleep, I couldn't believe it. A part of me was ready to accept that we might not make any real progress after following these protocols. But another part of me just kept saying, hang in there. Just have faith. It'll come.

As I continued to text with my mom about Ethan's progress, I reminded her that we were supposed to get him started on his new fish oil in just a few days.

"I started him on it the other day," she replied.

It was a little early, but it's not like there was a major issue with getting him started a few days ahead of schedule. And that's when it clicked. When I had spoken to SpeechNutrients about what response we might see from starting Ethan on their omega-3 supplement, they told me I could expect to see him have some sort of reaction at first, that he might act up a bit. They said that that was normal and it was actually a good sign. It meant that he was responding to it and that we would likely see him settle down soon after his body adjusted. So his excitement from the night we went to the farmer's market now made complete sense. It was his reaction to the fish oil. This left me even more excited about what would come next.

His sleep had improved, he had become more responsive, and he was starting to answer question in full sentences. *This* was major.

My mom continued to rave about how much more expressive he was. This was beyond motivating. We were seeing great progress and that silver lining was starting to shine even brighter.

A Shot of Hope

As my mom says, "Autism is like playing a sport. Some days you're sore and tired. Sometimes you feel like a champ. You make mistakes. You turn it around. You win some and lose some. At the end of it all there is a constant strive for victory . . . And you say, 'Damn, I love this life.'"

Here is my 1 in 68:

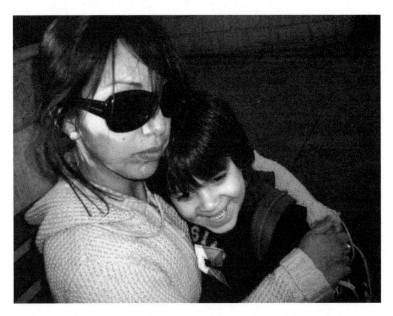

Never underestimate the power of a real mother warrior.

CHAPTER SEVENTEEN

The Light at the End of the Tunnel

The following month I was in Chicago for an autism benefit. It was an awesome annual event hosted by the parents of a child on the autism spectrum. With treatment, their child had improved significantly, and they made it their mission to give back to other families in need.

I was working the event and was really excited to be in town. I had been to Chicago and other parts of Illinois a few times, but this time I actually got to stay downtown.

The event was another great success. Lots of money was raised for charity, the sponsors were great, the people were great, and the food was delicious. Not that I was at all surprised.

The event always went well, and I was happy to be surrounded by such incredible people working so fiercely for a very worthy cause. The altruism in the room was inspiring.

After the event, my colleague Karen and I got stuck in Chicago for another night because we missed our flight, but this allowed us some nice bonding time. We had never had the chance to talk one-on-one. Karen is older than I am, and I've always looked up to her as a mentor. She's a brilliant woman who dedicates herself to her job and her family. And one thing we have in common is that we both have younger siblings with special needs.

Karen and I shared our experiences as older siblings pioneering the way for our younger siblings. We both felt that we were the ones who drove the recovery train when it came to our siblings, and we each shared a lot of the same feelings regarding the whole situation. I opened up to her about the struggle I've had with Ethan and with my family. It was really nice to have a real conversation with someone who genuinely understood where I was coming from. I had talked to friends and other colleagues, but never found someone who could relate to me in this way.

I often struggle with boundaries. How do I not step over the line with my mom? She's Ethan's parent, not me, so I have to be careful with how far I go with everything. But at the same time, I feel that if I'm not constantly bulldozing, Ethan's recovery might slip, which isn't fair to him. If that means having to constantly bulldoze, so be it. But at the same time, I would like to "retire" from autism at some point, or at least not have it consume 98 percent of my life. That's fair, right?

I keep waiting to reach the light at the end of the tunnel, but when and how do I get there? I get a glimpse of it every once in a while but then it fades. I just want to get there already and know that Ethan is in a really good place.

Ethan has improved so much with our recent attempt at biomed. He's making long strides toward a more independent life. He's in that preteen stage, so the hormones are starting to kick in, and the biomed treatment isn't quite as easy to apply as it was before. He's already set in some of his ways.

I have high hopes for a bright future. My original goal when writing this chapter was to say, "Yes, Ethan's fully recovered! We've reached the light at the end of the tunnel!" But for the longest time this chapter has remained pretty much blank except for my note: *Chapter still needs to be written.*

It was in Chicago with Karen that I realized the journey never really ends. There will always be struggles and milestones, but I'm not sure we'll reach the end of the tunnel, or if the damn tunnel even ends. Shit, for all I know, the lights I keep seeing might just be other trains heading in our direction, and success is somehow dodging them without getting killed. The thing is, I'm such a control freak that I like knowing all the answers and I like knowing when I reach my destination. But by missing our flight, I got to spend a nice night in a nice city and have a really nice conversation with a nice person. It forced me to be present and to not stress out or worry because, for once, things were not in my control.

As for Ethan and autism, I guess I've come to realize that the end result might not be in my control either. And maybe I have to stop worrying and just trust that I'm doing all that I can and hope for the best. I think, in some capacity, this is a small victory. This is the light in my tunnel. It's a torch that's helping me find my way. So, I really have nothing to complain about. I'm doing well, Ethan's making progress, and my family is doing better. Everything seems to be moving in the right direction. Something's got to be right. Right?

A Shot of Hope
Here is my recipe for the perfect "Light at the End of the Tunnel" cocktail:

1 shot of hope

Equal parts trust and instinct

1 ounce of courage (liquid substitute will suffice, if needed)

1 large helping of strength and tenacity

CHAPTER EIGHTEEN

Who Am I?

"So what's your story?" a new team member at my office once asked me.

Instantly my mind began racing. Normally I might answer this kind of question with, "My brother has autism," or talk about the work I do for autism. It's easy to tell my story that way.

I remember getting into a disagreement with a woman while working on a fund-raiser together. The event was cancelled days before its scheduled date because of a paperwork issue, and she was upset with the way I handled it. She even called me a "total narcissist."

"You're always talking about how in love with yourself you are," she barked.

"Oh, come on. You can't honestly think I'm serious? They're *jokes*. They're not meant to be taken seriously." About 99 percent of the comments I make are my attempts at being funny mainly because I really don't think all that highly of myself. Anybody who really knows me knows that I surely do lack confidence."

"Oh please. Nobody even knows you're a comedian," the woman responded. "All people know you as is the kid who wrote a book about his autistic brother."

Since that day, I've tried my best to fight that statement and prove that I am a lot more than that, that I am my own person with my own mind and voice, and that I am not defined by my brother's autism. Yes, it's something that has greatly impacted my life, but no, it is not something that I will let define me or my brother.

It isn't easy. My life is so centered on autism that no matter how hard I fight being labeled with it, there are days when I feel like maybe it is who I am. Every time *my story* comes up, it's still hard for me not to let autism come up. This has really made me think, outside of autism, what is my story? Who am I?

Finding my own identity has been one of the biggest struggles I've had to face. I was so young when I began my advocacy that I never expected my life to be so consumed by the cause. And the second I decided to start focusing on my own career goals, I still found them linking back to autism in some way.

When I began doing stand-up, I would do shows that benefited autism. I would use my humor in my books and in my speaking engagements, which, again, all linked back to autism. When I decided to develop my own liquor brand, I wanted to make sure the proceeds went back to autism. Everything was just *autism, autism, autism*. When your life becomes so overwhelmed with one subject, how do you move on from that subject? How do I move on from autism and not feel like the worst person in the world? Is it possible to be my own person at the same time? If so, *how*? My mind races with these questions daily.

I was out for coffee one day with my friend Deborah. She and I had met (surprise!) through autism. She ran a summer camp for kids with disabilities that Ethan had been attending. My mother thought it'd be best for me to volunteer my time there and act as Ethan's aid. Deb and I instantly hit it off. She loved trash TV just as much as I did, understood autism the way that I did, and was a chronic workaholic just as I am. Personality- and humor-wise, we're a lot alike. She gets me and I get her. But we're also complete opposites. She'll go out in sweatpants, a T-shirt, and a pair of furry slippers. I'll never leave the house in sweats and don't understand people who wear slippers outside (let alone ones with fur). She loves to shop at Walmart, and I can't stand the place (way too many crazies). And lastly, Deborah hates alcohol.

Now, fast-forward through all the charity-world drama, family drama, and many personal life crises, and ta-da, Deb and I are still friends. Despite how terrible I am at making friends (and even worse at keeping them), Deb and I have somehow managed through all the ups and downs over the years and still meet up regularly for our favorite meal of the day: coffee.

"I had a dream about you last night," Deborah told me. "It was, like, in the future. You were famous and I was trying to explain to these people that I knew you. I was like, 'The autism guy, yeah. I know him!'"

Listening to her describe me as "the autism guy" struck me the wrong way. Was that really how people were going to perceive me for the rest of my life? As it was, I've had swarms of trolls trying to make me feel bad for "exploiting" my brother and "using him." I am not trying to use him and I certainly don't want to exploit him. It's just that autism is such a big part of my life, and he's my connection to it. The opportunities I've gained through autism have helped me support his recovery. But at the same time, I'd still like to be just Zack, not the "autism guy."

When I first entered college, I was still pretty new to stand-up and learning to embrace my humor. I had met a group of people with whom I became very close. We would go out together and hang out at each other's houses. For once I was allowing myself to have a social life. I was allowing myself to actually have friends my age, instead of those twice my junior.

Looking back at that time now, I realized how much my attention was away from Ethan and my family. It's actually a period I felt guilty about for a long time. I was having fun being young and living my own life. It was probably the one year of my life that wasn't dominated by autism. I'll be honest, it felt free and liberating. I was focusing more time on building a career in entertainment rather than on autism. I was embracing friendship and even beginning to experience a little romance at the same time, which was something I never saw coming in a million years.

Well, before I knew it, the "friendships" started crumbling. Those who had once embraced me for my "Zack-ness" were now crucifying me, almost as if they were trying to find reasons to vote me off the island.

"What happened to all your friends?" my mom asked me around that time.

"I have friends," I told her.

"What happened to your Chinese friend and all the other friends you used to have?"

"I don't know," I replied, hoping to avoid the conversation.

"It might be good for you to go out and make some new friends. Experience life."

"I'm experiencing life, Mom. I'm just a little too busy to be worried about being the most popular person with lots of friends. I have friends. I just don't have time for lots of them."

In meeting many families affected by autism, I've found this to be common. Honestly, autism can become a full-time job. Recovery sure as hell isn't easy. It's something you have to stay dedicated to day after day.

I begin to think about what we would do if Ethan never gets to a point where he can live independently. Is anyone in my family even comfortable with allowing him to do that one day, given a full recovery? And if we're too overprotective, who's going to take care of him when he's older? Which brings us back to the question, when does autism end? Is it really a life-long disorder, not only for the individual diagnosed, but for everyone around him?

I've come across a few families that have reached recovery, or at least have reached a good level of progress. The second the autism dies down, they're ready to move on with their lives, which, in a way, frustrates me a little. I mean, they could use their testimonies to give hope to a newly diagnosed family. But is that really their responsibility? Do I wish they would stick around to help fight this battle? Yes. Do I blame them for trying to move on with their lives? No. I think everyone should be able to do that.

When it comes to Ethan, I want him to be able to live autism-free. I don't want him to have to feel limited because of a diagnosis. I want him to be just Ethan, not Ethan with autism. If he chooses to make autism part of his life, I'll fully support that. But I'd like him to have the choice.

The same goes for EJ, who lives with Ethan on a daily basis. I want him to live his life to the fullest and not have to worry about Ethan. I want him to be EJ, whomever he chooses to be. The same for my mom. I can see her maybe one day running her own little coffee shop decorated with the eccentric little knickknacks she loves.

As for me, I see myself owning my own home, feeling comfortable financially, but still working my ass off every day because I love it. And I still see autism being a part of my life but not so overbearing. I guess my mission is to do everything possible to help bring the numbers down and the severity down, or at least make treatment much more accessible and recovery rates much higher. Is that too optimistic? And maybe one day, autism won't have to be something that defines me, but something I *choose* to support.

I'm not the hero of this story, nor am I the villain. I'd prefer to be called a warrior or a fighter. Warriors have to take part in battles, and the only way to win is to give it all you've got.

So, who am I? It's plain and simple: I'm just a guy living his life. I'm fighting this battle for my family and trying to ensure my brother's independence. I like to give to myself just as much as I like to give to others. I am not defined by my job, my profession, or my surroundings. And I sure as hell am not defined by autism. I'm just plain old Zack.

A Shot of Hope

As people, we grow and we mature unless we make the decision to stay the same. But the choice is all yours. Do you know who *you* are?

Sidenote: When I finished this chapter and headed back up to my hotel room, I happened to overhear a man talking about his nephew with autism. I told you, not a day goes by without hearing that word.

The Hope Rules

L ife can be a shit storm of misery or a basket of bless-
ings—it really depends on how you look at it. It's easy
to fall into the "woe is me" pit. I mean, come on, I love
a good pity party as much as the next person. But after the
first five minutes, you need to move on. That's a lesson I've
learned.

I've learned that sometimes you just have to keep pushing
through it. It always gets better. Sometimes it gets worse, but
usually after that it gets better. You just have to have hope.

What is hope? I use the word a lot. To me, hope is seeing
potential, believing in it, and being willing to work your ass
off to reach it. It's opportunity. To have hope means to see
the end result and to desperately want it and also be willing to work for it. If someone had come to me when I was

twelve years old and told me that my brother's diagnosis would motivate me to become an empowered and dedicated young adult, I would've laughed and said, "Yeah, right." Yet, here I am, writing my fourth book about how I got here. And it was all due to hope. Hope is not just the *want*; it's also the willingness to take action, to get up and *do something.* That's hope.

This journey with Ethan, with my family, and with myself has been nothing short of a wild ride. It's taught me so much. I want people to feel empowered and motivated so that even when they get knocked down, they'll get back up and keep fighting.

Along the way, I've compiled this list of rules. It's a list of reminders that I use to help me hold my head up when I feel my hope slipping. I call them the Hope Rules. They're something to work at every day. Some days some rules are more important than others. Some days, I say fuck it and disregard them altogether. Hopefully they'll help you too.

1. Know Yourself; Know Your Mission

This is a rule of truth. I don't believe a person can ever entirely know himself, but there are certain traits we can be pretty certain about (though there are times when we surprise ourselves).

It's really all about knowing what you want. If you don't know who the hell you are, how can you know where the hell to go? And if you don't know where you want to go, how are you supposed to get there?

2. Take the Cards Life Gives You, but Never Settle for Them

People tend to think "acceptance" means "settling." There's a big difference. I don't know how many times I've seen "F that" on Facebook following the topic of acceptance for autism. I'm going to start off by telling you that bitterness won't get you anywhere and this attitude won't either.

Acceptance *is* the key to opening doors, especially when it comes to autism recovery. Now, I'm not telling you to accept that life will be like this forever, but you do need to accept that there has been a diagnosis and that autism is now in your life. You have to realize that the course you were previously on is no longer the course in front of you. You can't be pissed about the cards life deals you and just throw them up in the air and walk out. Life doesn't work that way. You have to accept the hand you've been dealt and play the game to your advantage.

Acceptance doesn't mean the world is over. It's not a closed door. It's a brand-new door opening onto a world of possibilities. There are only two doors. One is acceptance and the other is settling. One door leads to hope and the other leads to bitter submission. The choice is yours. But if you want my two cents' worth, I'd suggest you don't settle.

3. Challenge Yourself and Never Stop Pushing

I've found that the risks I've taken have always scared the shit out of me at first. Fear is probably one of the greatest motivators. As long as it keeps you on your toes, makes you a little excited, it's probably the right thing.

Now, I'm not telling you to jump off a cliff and try to make yourself invincible. Clearly you need to have some discretion and not be reckless. But challenge yourself. It's how you grow. By challenging myself, I've been able to gain so much strength, mostly inner strength. If you've seen my scrawny body, you'll know there's not much physical strength going on there.

4. Never Hope for It More than You're Willing to Work for It

Hope is extremely important, but so is hard work. If you're not willing to get your hands dirty and work hard toward your goal, you'll never reach it. That's just the reality. Hope is vital, but at the end of the day, hope is just hope. Hope is not action. You must take action along with hope. All I can do is share my experience and give you a little motivation to keep going. I can give you the tools that I've found helpful, but unless you're willing to actually put them into effect, you're not going to get anywhere.

I candidly wrote about Ethan's regression and how much guilt I had over it. The main reason I felt guilty was because I had stopped working toward his recovery. His treatment protocol wasn't in effect; therefore, he wasn't seeing any progress. This taught me the importance of this rule. You can wish for something to come true, but unless you do something about it, you can kiss that wish good-bye! Your hope should always be as strong as your attempt and vice versa. You're not going to get very far without both being fully charged.

So, basically this rule is: Get your ass off the couch and get to work!

5. A Hustler's Work Never Ends, so Make Sure to Work Hard, Play Hard, *and* Rest Hard

This is one of my favorite rules. Normally, the advice is *work hard, play hard*. But there's just one little piece that gets left out and that's *rest hard*. Taking care of yourself is one of the most important things you need to do for your sanity and overall well-being.

One of the most important lessons I've learned over the years is that self-care is crucial. I was taking on heavy workloads at a very young age, in addition to going to school full-time. Eventually it caught up to me. I remember having anxiety attacks, one while I was in class. Luckily it was in history class and the teacher was a total bore, but the reality is, someone my age should not be having anxiety attacks.

So, this is how I like to handle this rule. Monday through Friday, I work hard. Friday evenings and Saturdays are for having fun and playing hard. And Sundays are for resting hard.

6. Remember the Destination and Appreciate the Process

So many times I've found myself focusing on how hard it is and how far I feel like I still have to go that I forget about the destination. Like with Ethan, sometimes I worry about him not doing well in the moment and automatically assume the worst. My thoughts just start building up with anxiety and before I know it, my imagination has me losing an arm or leg in a freak car accident so that I'm unable to assist Ethan when he's older.

Anyway, my point is that oftentimes I allow fear of what might come get in the way of just trusting that everything happens for a reason and every challenge will bring some sort of strength or clarity. This is why it's important to just appreciate what is and accept the process but never forget the destination. That's the part that's going to keep you motivated. If you forget where you're trying to go, you'll get lost.

7. Ain't Nobody Got Time for That Negative Bullshit
Inspired by Sweet Brown, this is a very important rule for staying sane and dignified. I am all for a good, nourishing debate. I think debate is important and as long as you go in with genuine passion and a listening ear, both parties can really thrive from it. However, you need to know when to back off from the crazies and negative trolls. People like to fight. Fighting is pointless. If there are people in your life who are creating a negative environment, they're toxic and should be removed. This includes trolls on the Internet, media bullies, and even people in your everyday life.

I've been in several situations where I was around the wrong people. I once had a friend who seemed like a very cool person to hang out with. However, I started to notice that every single time we went out, I always treated, or that when I needed his friendship, he'd be there only when it was convenient for him. Then I realized, why am I complaining about this situation, when I can clearly resolve it? And I did.

Negative people draw only negative results. Toxic people create only toxic surroundings. Draining people just drain you. How can you fulfill your personal mission if your focus is in the wrong place with the wrong people? Life is way too damn short to be with people who bring you down.

The same thing applies when you put your focus in the wrong place. Yes, focus on the positive, but make sure that the focus is on *your* positive. Not someone else's "happy life." The grass is never greener on the other side. It is especially crucial in the autism community. When I saw other people having success with their kids, I would take my focus away from Ethan's progress. That wasn't fair to me or him. The focus needs to be in the right place.

8. Never End the Day unless It's Productive

The only way I allow myself to go to bed satisfied is when I ask myself, "Did I kick ass today?" and the answer is yes. Kicking ass doesn't always mean being Superman and saving kids from burning buildings. Sometimes, it just means making it through the day without jumping out the window. I mean, some days I just can't put out every single fire that comes my way, but just making it through without letting the fire burn me to ashes is an accomplishment.

I'll tell you right now, you're a total badass. Everybody has the potential to be. Just believe in yourself. And give it your best shot. If you can say you've definitely given it your best shot, then at the end of the day, you're fully entitled to enjoy a shot of vodka to go with your shot of hope.

9. ALWAYS STAY Benefi+

I like to live according to what I consider the "Benefi+" lifestyle. Benefi+ is a lifestyle brand I developed that shares my philosophy of giving. Give to others and give to yourself.

Be good to people around you, and at the same time remember to nourish yourself. Whether it be with the food you eat or the activities you participate in or the knowledge you strive to gain, try to make sure that it's not only healthy for you, but also good for others. Lead a life with meaning, while also taking care of yourself.

Staying Benefi+ is not, however, to be confused with idealism or perfectionism. Giving, no matter how large or small, creates a better environment for us all. Try to improve yourself and try to improve circumstances for others as well. Some people may think, *Well, that's not my responsibility.* You're right; it's not. But what if you were in a rut and someone came to help you? Think how much greater this world would be if we all simply just paid it forward once in a while.

10. Laugh

Ah, alas, the final rule. When you've made it through the day, kicked ass, stayed focused, and reached some progress, enjoy it. People always wonder how I can joke and poke fun at everything in my life. It's easy. I need to.

If I didn't make fun of things, I would be suicidal. I would literally want to shoot myself in the face if I couldn't laugh. Lots of people will say that autism is such a serious topic, there's not room for humor. And I laugh at them. I laugh because that's such a sad outlook on life. I want nothing to do with that. I want to live my life to the fullest, enjoy it, and laugh about it.

Look back at whatever drives you crazy, and just laugh about it.

Recently, my mom told me that Ethan's therapist was over at the house and he asked Ethan a bunch of questions.

"What does Mom like to eat?" he asked.

"Food," Ethan said.

"What does Mom like to drink?"

"Beer!" Ethan exclaimed.

Some people might find that offensive or inappropriate. We just laugh.

A Shot of Hope

I just gave you my ten rules for keeping your hope strong, while still maintaining your dignity and sanity. Do you really need more from me?

Inside the Mind of an Autism Sibling

I get asked questions all the time about what it's like to be a sibling of someone with autism. And most of the time, the questions are usually the same. So I took the liberty to answer them in an open Q&A here. You're welcome.

Q: What's it like being a sibling of someone with autism?

Zack: Well, do *you* have a sibling? It's kind of like that. I have a total of six younger siblings. (Yeah, apparently my parents didn't have much else to do.) Only one has autism. I don't really know how Ethan is any more or less important than the others. Of all of them, he's just the one who's required more of my attention because of his special needs that we've had to address. It's difficult at times, yes. It's frustrating. I guess the best way I can describe it is that it's like receiving a gift on Christmas. Now pretend you already know exactly what that gift is going to be. You have a very clear idea of it in your head. Then, on Christmas morning when you open the gift, it's exactly what you were expecting. But then it turns out to be something different from what you thought it was going to be. Not necessarily better or worse, just different. So then you just have to adapt to it. For anybody who has more than one sibling or more than one child, have they all been exactly the same? *No.* They're all different. Each one has his and her own needs and eccentricities. So you treat each one as an individual. Some come with more challenges and some are more easygoing. Ethan just happened to come with a few more challenges than we expected. So to answer that question: It's a little more challenging, but equally rewarding. He's still my little brother, nonetheless.

Q: Is it hard having a brother with autism?

Zack: A lot of things are hard. If I sat around all day and counted how many difficulties I've faced in my life, I'd be depressed and unable to function. Yes, it's difficult at times. But I like to focus more on the rewards that come after each obstacle. And I like to look back and laugh about the hardships we've overcome together. It's really taught me how to have a sense of humor.

Q: What do you love about your brother?

Zack: I think this is probably one of the questions I like the least. For me to have to think of one thing I love about my brother just seems so asinine to me. How do you pick one thing? I don't like having to think of a reason to love someone. It's just an innate love that you have for people. There's no *one* thing that I love about my brother. I just love my brother. He's special and unique in his own way, and I love him for that.

Q: How can I get my kid to be more like you?

Zack: Trust me, the last thing you want is for your kid to be more like me! I'm a little too honest, a bit of a control freak, and one of the biggest workaholics you'll come across. My emotional turmoil is through the roof! Let's just say, I'm a bit of a mess. But if you want your kids to be proactive, I'd suggest just supporting them in anything and everything they want. Support them, encourage them, love them. But don't baby them or push them too hard. You want them to be self-sufficient and independent. Only you know where that line is with your child.

Q: How do I reach my kids without autism?

Zack: Try texting them. I'm sure that'll work. They're probably on their phones 24-7, am I right? I'm kidding. I'd say the best way to reach them would be by allowing them in. Sometimes I think parents are too absorbed in autism that they forget to pay attention to their kids without autism. And most times, the extra responsibility is assumed by the siblings. Just be sure to appreciate them, let them know you're there for them too, and have open conversations with them. They need that. Make them feel included. Without that, they'll likely feel lost and left out, which is *no bueno.*

Q: What's the best advice you'd give to a parent managing a household that includes a child with special needs?

Zack: Make sure you let your other kids know they're acknowledged. The one piece of advice I always give to parents is to make sure you set aside time for them too. Whether it's once a week or once a month, just let them know that they have your undivided attention. Make it a day out. Whatever it is, just make sure you have some time set aside for them to feel important too. And whatever you do, please, please, please just keep the date. Don't cancel it. It'll crush your kids. It crushed me every single time.

Q: What advice would you give to a fellow sibling?

Zack: Hang in there. I could go on and on about what I would tell siblings, but the short answer is: *hang in there.* Help out as much as you can. It'll get better, I promise.

Q: You have so much going on at such a young age. How do you do it?

Zack: This is another question that's so common and oh so tough to answer. There's really no answer to that. It's just my life. It's not always easy and nothing's ever perfectly balanced. Some things fall as others rise. Not everything is always great, and not everything is always terrible. I just take it one day at a time, sometimes one hour at a time with lots of coffee in between. And vodka. I think that's my secret: coffee and vodka. One time I even mixed the two of them together. I don't recommend doing that.

Now anytime someone asks me one of these questions, I will refer them to this chapter. So if you happen to ask me any of these, just a warning. I will simply reply, "Buy my book. That's why I wrote it."

Some Words of Advice to My Fellow Siblings

I am the oldest of seven kids. "Sibling" would definitely count as just one of the many titles I try to juggle on a daily basis. To be quite honest, I think it's one of the most defining. Especially being the oldest. I constantly feel responsible for my brothers and sister. I may not always show it, but their well-being always trumps mine. Or at least I try to always put it before mine. I know some might argue that that might not be the healthiest thing to do, but it's just who I am.

I look at Ethan no differently than I look at the other five of them. He is just as much a blessing as he is a pain in the butt. He's the little brother who makes me laugh, and he's the little brother who makes me want to pull my hair out. Autism or not, he's still my brother.

I look at my other brother EJ and at times, my stomach hurts. I see a young boy growing into a young man at a rapid rate. I see him struggling to find his identity as the middle child. "People always ask what's it like to be Ethan's brother, or what it's like to be Zack's brother," he said once, and it struck a nerve with me. Ethan and I never intentionally try to take the spotlight away from him; we just naturally demand more attention. Ethan needs the extra attention, and I have so much going on in my life that it often draws people's eyes in my direction. And on the flip side of things, I look at EJ at times and I think, *Wow, that's one badass kid.* Sure, he has a mouth on him and an even bigger attitude, but at his age, which one of us didn't? I look at him, and at how much fun he still has at his age despite all the challenges life's thrown his way. I never wanted him or Ethan to have to experience what it's like to live in two different households. I never wanted EJ to have to assume the extra responsibility of Ethan. I never wanted him to feel on his own. I'll be the first to admit, I've given more of my devotion to Ethan than I have to EJ. And for that, I do apologize. I can't take any of that lost time back, but going forward, I can make sure that EJ knows that I am there for him, no matter what. All I can be at this point is the best big brother I know how to be. I didn't have any older siblings, so I don't really have a model to follow, but I can be an example for all the little ones.

I look at my siblings on my father's side and thank God every day that they still have a strong and stable household. I've chosen to not name any of them in this book to protect their privacy. They're not exactly part of this journey with autism but have still been supportive. For that, I am thankful.

If there are any words of encouragement I can give you, whether you're struggling to accept that autism is now in your family or facing any of the struggles I've openly discussed in this book, I would start with: Take it all one day at a time. Breathe. It gets better.

It's hard. There's no sugarcoating it. It's really hard. It sucks. It hurts. At times, it's lonely. The spotlight is pulled from you and you're left in the dark. I understand it. I've felt it all. I've been frustrated with my family. I've been frustrated with myself. If there's any guilt you have, it's time to let it go. Stop blaming yourself. Allow yourself to hurt. Allow yourself to get mad. Let it out. The more you hold it in, the more it's going to dig deeply inside you and begin changing the person you thought you knew.

Start talking about it. Talk to your parents. Talk to friends. Talk to someone. Write if you need to. Let it out. Find a way to let out the emotions you're trying to bottle up. You may feel weak, but you're far stronger than you ever thought.

The reality of what the future may hold is still undetermined, so stop making it up in your head. Work hard every single day and trust that it'll work out.

Your parents need you right now. And the truth is, you need them a whole lot more, which is why you need to lean on each other. Be a family. That's the only way to beat the harsh brutality that comes with autism. The world you thought you knew just got rattled, and the only way you're going to stay standing up straight is with the help of a strong team. That team is your family.

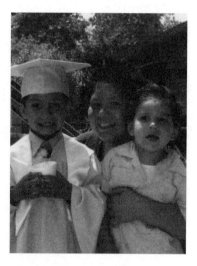

Don't take anything personally. I took a lot personally when I was growing up. But I learned that people are struggling every day. They act out because they get tired of

EJ, me, Deets.

being strong on their own. Let them know they don't have to

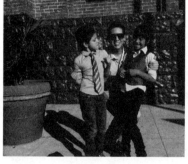

Oh, you know, brothers just striking a pose . . .

be. If it's your siblings, be there for them. If it's your parents, support them.

When it comes to your friends, some of them won't like that you have a brother or sister with autism. Let them go. Kick them out of your life as soon as possible. Keep only the people who are going to help you grow, who are going to help you and your family. When you find them, keep them close.

Other Little Shots of Hope

Here are more little shots of hope that should help motivate you. Or at least give you a little laugh to make it through the day.

Always carry a fire extinguisher. You never know when you'll need to put out a fire. If your life is anything like mine, it's daily. Be prepared.

Persistence and determination will get you everything you could ever need. So always follow your hunch.

Candor is important. You should always speak your mind and be as honest about what you want as possible. I always say, "Never beat around the bush."

If plans don't work out as anticipated, that's okay. Think of them like your exes: you didn't want them anyway!

Life can be unpredictable. Trying to keep your balance is tough (especially after the third margarita). Just hold your head up and keep walking. Crawl if you must. Just don't stop moving.

When life hands you lemons, throw them at people! Just make sure they're the right people.

Don't take anything (especially yourself) too seriously. That's just annoying for everyone.

Never settle. When you settle, you give up on yourself. When you give up on yourself, you end up with someone like Kevin Federline.

When traveling with my mother, always make sure she's not in charge of making the arrangements.

Remember, there's no such thing as false hope. And anybody who tries to argue is simply a troll. Trolls are not worth the time of day.

Above all, never give up.

Dear Deets . . .

In my first book, I had an entire chapter made up of diary entries I had written to Ethan when I was fifteen. People appreciated it so much because it really let them not only into my mind but also into my heart. So, here's my last diary entry to Ethan. It's my last one because from here on out, I will no longer be writing diary entries for Ethan to read *one day*. Starting *today*, I will begin having small conversations with Ethan. And, in time, we will have full-on conversations. I am certain of it. We're already getting there . . .

Dear Deets,

Where do I even begin? You're twelve now. I'm twenty-one. It's been such an adventure. Me, you, Mom, EJ, your dad, everyone—we've all come so far. And we've all gotten the chance to watch you come so far. Watching you reach milestones brings so much excitement to my life. I've learned how to really appreciate the things that matter in life because of you. I look at the things we often take for granted and I've come to hold them as so much more sacred. I pray for you every day. I want you to know that. I pray for strength and energy . . . and that there's never a coffee shortage. One day, you're going to make fun of me for all the coffee I drink. And for the fact that I drink it with a straw to keep my teeth white. And I'll say, "Oh, shut up, Deets," as a big brother should. And I'll also be there when times get tough. And I'll say, "It'll be okay, Deeties." I look forward to all these conversations we'll have one day. This will all be worth it. I know it will . . . But until then, I'm just going to work my ass off and keep fighting until we finally reach that day. I'll see you on the other end!

Thank you,
Zack

Epilogue: Saving Deets

I titled the very first book I wrote *Saving Deets*. That's originally what my story was about: saving my brother from the cruelty and ridicule of this world, from having to live a life reliant on other people, and from not being able to have the future he chooses to have. But along the way, I've learned so much that I feel like he's saved me a lot more than I've saved him. And that's been my journey: finding myself in helping my brother.

I've had people tell me over the years, "One day, Deets is going to thank you for all you do for him." It always makes me a little emotional hearing that. Ethan has changed my life in so many ways, I don't even know where to begin. And I can't wait for the day I really get to *thank him*.

I often question why I was given this life. Sometimes I'm just like, "What could I have possibly done in a previous life that would have thrust such an adventure onto me now?" I'm still figuring that out.

But what I do know is that I'm coming out of this so much stronger. My relationship with my family is so much better. Ethan is doing great! He's more responsive and more expressive. He's sleeping so much better! Dr. Jerry has been guiding us through everything and everyone's on board and doing their part. Everything is just really falling into place. But I'm sure there are likely to be more bumps in the road as there have been many times before. But I feel like I'm ready for whatever life throws at us next.

I hope that by sharing my story with you, you've learned a thing or two. Whether it's that there really is hope for autism or that I've had some really bad travel experiences, I hope that you take something away from it like a little motivation, a few laughs, and a shot or two of hope!

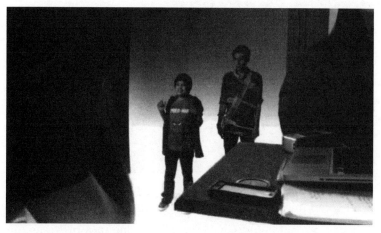

A real little superhero right here, working hard every day. (Yeah, he tied me up in caution tape. It was his form of a disclaimer.)

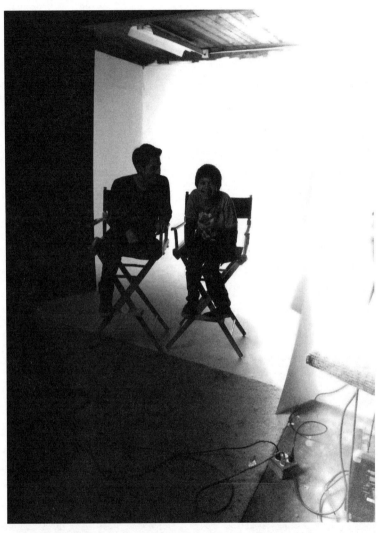

Me and Deets—the future sure does look bright for us!

Resources

Here's a list of some of my favorite go-to resources that were a huge help when it came to writing this book and healing Ethan's autism. I hope you find these resources as helpful as I did. Without them, I would really be lost.

Websites/Blogs

Mending Autism
www.mendingautism.com

This is Dr. Jerry Kartzinel's blog. It has so much information and it's all so easy to grasp.

Generation Rescue
www.generationrescue.org

I'm on this site daily. There is so much information not just on treatment, but also on recovery updates, great products, steps new parents can take to prevent autism, and helpful links to other resources.

Environmental Working Group
www.ewg.org

This site is a nontoxic lifesaver! I research all of my personal and household cleaning products through them. I use their site and their iPhone apps. Such a great resource!

Healthy Child Healthy World
www.healthychildhealthyworld.org

This site is great for parents looking to raise healthy kids in this toxic world. They have so many great articles and links to some of their trusted products, which I found really came in handy!

Products

Sunlighten Saunas
www.sunlighten.com

They have some of the best infrared saunas available for healthy detox! This was crucial in helping Ethan get everyday toxins and heavy metals out of his body. And it was great for calming him down before bed.

IntelliBED

www.intellibed.com

This company has been amazing to my family. I've had such awesome calls with them about nontoxic sleep and the importance of a quality mattress. You'd be surprised about the toxins you're sleeping on!

The Honest Company

www.honest.com

I have their monthly bundle package. Their nontoxic cleaning products are the best. I've converted so many people that I've considered taking up Scientology because of how great I am at it.

SpeechNutrients

www.speechnutrients.com

Another great company. Ethan takes their omega-3 capsules. He had a hard time with taking liquid fish oils, but these were great. Awesome quality.

Kartzinel Health

www.kartzinelhealth.com

Ethan and I take Dr. Jerry's multivitamin capsules, which have led to great results! I used to take a gummy multivitamin, which never gave me the boost that these do. The Kartzinel line is exceptional.

Enzymedica
www.enzymedica.com

Amazing digestive enzymes for just about everything. Ethan
and I take their Digestive Spectrum capsules.

BioRay
www.bioray.com

Great products for healthy detox and repairing the GI tract.
Ethan is on a couple of their products, which have led to
great results.

Books

The Honest Life: Living Naturally and True to You by
Jessica Alba
   A great guidebook to nontoxic living. I know, it's a celebrity
book, so how much credibility can it really have? Trust me, it's
a good read. Lots of great information!

Healing and Preventing Autism: A Complete Guide by Jenny
McCarthy and Jerry Kartzinel, MD
   I live by this book. I've read it so many times. It's a great
resource for all of your healing autism questions.

*The Autism Book: What Every Parent Needs to Know about
Early Detection, Treatment, Recovery, and Prevention* by
Robert W. Sears, MD, FAAP

Dr. Sears is great. He always has very helpful information in his books.

The Vaccine Book: Making the Right Decision for Your Child by Robert W. Sears, MD, FAAP

A very good, unbiased look at vaccines, both the pros and the cons. This is a great book for someone looking to make an informed decision.

Evidence of Harm: Mercury in Vaccines and the Autism Epidemic by David Kirby

There's a lot of good information in this one. It's very long and took me a while to get through, but it's a good read.

Nourishing Hope for Autism: Nutrition and Diet Guide for Healing Our Children by Julie Matthews

Julie Matthews is such an educated woman. She has such a dedication to health. Her books and website are great resources for the benefits of a simple change in diet.

Acknowledgments

Where do I start?

I want to thank an incredible boy named Ethan for kicking off this journey and helping me become the person I am today. I've learned so much from you, it's ridiculous. You, EJ, Shawn, Isaiah, Breanne, and Joshua have all made me such a better person, I love you all. I want to thank my mother, Nancy. Mom, you're beautiful inside and out and you always know how to keep me motivated. What would I do without you? (Just please try to work on your time management skills.)

My family, I love you all dearly. Thank you for all of the support over the years. And thank you for believing in me, especially at the times I found it hard to keep believing in myself.

A very special thank you to Candace McDonald, Stephanie Rotondi, and then entire Generation Rescue team. Working with you has been such a privilege. You've taught me so much and been amazing to me and my family. I am forever indebted to you.

Thank you Dr. Jerry Kartzinel, David, and the rest of the Kartzinel Wellness staff. You've been incredible with my brother and I am so thankful for everything you've done.

Deborah Noonan--what the hell would I do without you? Not only did you play a great role in helping me with this book, you've been an amazing friend.

Thank YOU, the reader. And to the brave warrior parents out there fighting for your kiddos. I've learned so much from you all. Thank you.

And, of course, thank you to Tony Lyons, Niels Aaboe, and the entire Skyhorse/Carrel Books team. Thank you for giving me a shot and putting up with me throughout this whole process. I was just a kid with a smart mouth and a story to tell. Thank you for allowing me tell that story.